SHARING MILK

BRISTOL
UNIVERSITY
PRESS

Gender and Sociology series

Series editors: **Sue Scott**, Newcastle University and **Stevi Jackson**, Centre for Women's Studies, University of York

---

Presenting high-quality research from established scholars and early-career researchers, the *Gender and Sociology* series is aimed at an international audience of academics and students who are interested in gender across the social science disciplines, particularly in sociology.

Forthcoming in the series:

Feminist Politics in Neoconservative Russia
An Ethnography of Feminist Resistance and Resources
Inna Perheentupa

Politicizing Childcare
Maternal Workers, Class and Contemporary Feminism
Maud Perrier

Chinese Men's Practices of Intimacy, Embodiment and Kinship
Crafting Elastic Masculinity
Siyang Cao

Austerity, Women and the Role of the State
Lived Experiences of the Crisis
Vicki Dabrowski

Out now in the series:

Work, Labour and Cleaning
The Social Contexts of Outsourcing Housework
Lotika Singha

Find out more at

bristoluniversitypress.co.uk/gender-and-sociology

Gender and Sociology series

Series editors: **Sue Scott**, Newcastle University and **Stevi Jackson**, Centre for Women's Studies, University of York

---

Presenting high-quality research from established scholars and early-career researchers, the *Gender and Sociology* series is aimed at an international audience of academics and students who are interested in gender across the social science disciplines, particularly in sociology.

International advisory board:

SHARING MILK

Intimacy, Materiality and Bio-Communities of Practice

Shannon K. Carter and
Beatriz M. Reyes-Foster

BRISTOL
UNIVERSITY
PRESS

First published in Great Britain in 2020 by

Bristol University Press
University of Bristol
1-9 Old Park Hill
Bristol
BS2 8BB
UK
t: +44 (0)117 954 5940
e: bup-info@bristol.ac.uk

Details of international sales and distribution partners are available at
bristoluniversitypress.co.uk

British Library Cataloguing in Publication Data
A catalogue record for this book is available from the British Library

ISBN 978-1-5292-0208-3 hardcover
ISBN 978-1-5292-0211-3 ePub
ISBN 978-1-5292-0209-0 ePdf

Cover design by blu inc, Bristol
Front cover image: urbazon – istockphoto.com
Bristol University Press uses environmentally responsible print partners
Printed and bound in Great Britain by CPI Group (UK) Ltd, Croydon, CR0 4YY

FSC
www.fsc.org
MIX
Paper from responsible sources
FSC® C013604

For milk sharers across the world

Contents

List of Figures and Tables

Figures

Tables

Notes on the Authors

Shannon K. Carter is a sociologist, professor and mother. Her research focuses on the ways social inequalities manifest in reproductive health and healthcare. She has published many articles on pregnancy, birth, breastfeeding and peer milk sharing in academic journals such as *Sociology of Health & Illness*, *Sociology of Race & Ethnicity*, *Breastfeeding Medicine* and *Gender & Society*. Her current research endeavours focus on reproductive healthcare experiences of individuals who identify as transgender and gender nonbinary, and birth in the US during the COVID-19 pandemic.

Beatriz M. Reyes-Foster is a medical anthropologist, author and mother. Her research interests focus on the interactions between individual actors and the medical and social structures they inhabit across a variety of contexts, including mental health care services in Mexico and reproductive health in the US. She is the author of *Psychiatric Encounters: Madness and Modernity in Yucatán, Mexico* (2018, Rutgers University Press). Alongside long-time collaborator Shannon Carter, she has published numerous articles on human milk sharing practices in the US.

Acknowledgements

This book is the product of the efforts and labour of many people. To begin with, this book would not have been possible without the milk-sharing parents and caretakers who generously agreed to participate in our research. We are grateful for the support of Sue Scott and Stevi Jackson, who believed in this book and made its publication possible. Shannon Kneis and Victoria Pittman at Bristol University Press have been instrumental in facilitating the reviews, revisions and production of this book. Three anonymous reviewers provided valuable feedback that greatly strengthened this manuscript. Kristin Wilson and Rhonda Shaw generously read and commented on parts of earlier versions of the manuscript. The Department of Sociology at the University of Central Florida provided funding to support data collection. The Gloria Anzaldúa Research Excellence Award by the Department of Women and Gender Studies at the University of Central Florida (UCF) provided support for images and dissemination. We thank our department Chairs, Libby Mustaine, John Schultz and Tosha Dupras, for their professional support during this process, as well as MC Santana of the Women and Gender Studies programme. We also thank Ajha Avin, Nicholas Boyce, Raquel Canepa, Kiana Cruz, Sarah Daabies, Lauren Daniel, Mariah Deremo, Erin Detzel, Kelly Gill, Cristina Hyman, Madeline Klayman, Katie Lamar, Estefany Londoño, Jenna McKelvey, Africa Pannozzi, Jennie St. Hilaire, Emma Tukdarian, Glenda Vaillant-Cruz and Julie Wynn for their assistance at various stages of research and writing. Earlier versions of this work were presented at the American Sociological Association annual meetings and the American Anthropological Association annual meetings, as well as the Southern Sociological Society conference, the Sociologists for Women in Society conference, the Motherhood conference, and the Central Florida Anthropological Society.

This work would not have been possible without the support of key members of the birth, breastfeeding and milk-sharing communities in Central Florida and beyond. Allika Alce-Garries, Becca Barnes, Chelsea

Bossory, Alejandra DeMaio, Heather Dunn, Crystal Fedele, Michelle Graf-Dixon, Michelle Isla, Alyssa Kaplan, Emma Kwasnica, Rebecca Luckey, Kelly Martin, Dee Mixer, Amanda Pacheco, Kaleen Richards, Alison Rockwell, Brooke Simmons, Natacha Soares Carreiro, Erin Spaulding, Morgan Thocher, Lora Vail and Angela Ziegler provided essential support and assistance that made this project possible. The Breastfeeding Project was immensely helpful in plugging us into the breastfeeding communities of Central Florida, and we are grateful for the various board members who served the organization, including Karen Andriola, Hollie Binette, Nichole Robins-Bowling, Jennifer Branting, Alexis Jetton-Galerno, Colleen Juul, Shawna Mitchell, Amanda Mulkey, Christina Rice, Emily Rupp, Brooke Taylor and Donna Urbina.

Shannon would like to thank the colleagues, friends and family members who supported this project. Many colleagues facilitated this book through conversations about the research, collaborations and feedback at conferences, including Katie Acosta, Mandi Barringer, Marni Brown, Anne Bubriski, David Embrick, Stephanie Gonzalez-Guittar, Liz Grauerholz, Melanie Hinojosa, April Hovav, Katie Johnson, Amanda Koontz, Tanya Koropeckyj-Cox, Nik Lampe, Cameron Lippard, Emily Mann, Susan Markens, Theresa Morris, Nicole Owens, Kylie Parrotta, Louise Roth, Brenda Savage, Carrie Lee Smith, Bhoomi Thakore, Angela Vergara, Miranda Waggoner and Elizabeth Ziff. I am particularly grateful for guidance and support from Sara Crawley. Colleagues I haven't met but interact with online also had an impact on the research, including Karleen Gribble, Aunchalee Palmquist, EA Quinn and Cecilia Tomori. I would also like to thank my friends who provided support and encouragement, especially Kelly Aissen, Natalie Arteaga, Melissa Bardwell, Stephanie Commings, Brad Darling, Julie Darling, Kari Day, Todd Day, Dana Gimeno, Brooke Haygood, Stacey Martindale, Rachel Royal and Chera Tramontin. I would like to acknowledge members of my family who have talked through this research with me for several years, especially Dan, Jan, Shawn, Maryann, Andrew, Matthew and Daniel Lawrence, as well as Irene Hagen and Lyssi Antrim. This work would not be possible without the assistance of my mom, Terry Lawrence, and my mother-in-law, Claudia Carter, who care for our children during conferences and other critical times during the academic year. Most of all, I am grateful for my children, Joshua, Ella and Auguste, who made my journey into motherhood and milk-sharing not only possible but amazing, and my husband Scott, who has always supported me as a mother and scholar.

Beatriz would like to offer thanks to many friends and colleagues at UCF and beyond. At UCF, Stacy Barber, Nessette Falu, Sandra Wheeler, and Lana Williams all provided helpful insight during lively discussions of our research. I am also grateful for the friendship of Crystle Bechtold, Amanda Major, Ilenia Colon Mendoza, Cecilia Milanes and Wanda Raimundi-Ortiz. Adrienne Pine was a wonderful collaborator, co-organizing a provocative and memorable panel at the American Anthropological Association annual meetings. I would also like to thank Aunchalee Palmquist, EA Quinn and Cecilia Tomori for their collegiality and insight over the years. My doula, Chylain Krivensky, was a close ally and confidant during the period where my personal and research lives blended and I navigated the difficulties of insufficient milk production. I would like to once again thank our donor, Heather Rich, for providing vital nutrition for our son in his first year. I am forever grateful for your selflessness and dedication, which has benefitted many babies, including my own, and helped me continue my breastfeeding journey in the face of many challenges. I thank my mother, Beatriz Cortes, for taking in stride my choice to feed my baby donor milk and revealing a family story I had been unaware of, that my great-grandmother frequently nursed her neighbours' babies in early 20th-century Mexico. My cousin, Brenda Valdez Hernandez, provided badly needed infant care during the data collection period of our research. Finally, I offer my deepest gratitude to my spouse, Ron Reyes-Foster, whose support was instrumental in giving me the time and space necessary to devote to this book, and to my children, Aydin, Rowan and Miles Reyes-Foster, who always keep my feet on the ground.

Preface

We are very pleased to have this book in a series that aims to bring original sociological thinking to bear on contemporary gender relations, divisions and issues of concern to feminists. It is our aim for the series that it will challenge received wisdom, offer new insights and expand the scope of sociology both theoretically and substantively.

We confess that milk sharing is a topic that we had not thought about sociologically prior to receiving the proposal from the authors of this book. Also, as non-mothers, it was not something we had encountered in our personal lives. However, this series seeks to embrace all aspects of gendered social life using sociological perspectives, and as it is one of the core aims of sociology to render the familiar strange and the unfamiliar comprehensible, and, as feeding infants is a significant area of many women's everyday lives we felt that the book was a good fit. The book illustrates the ways in which milk sharing disrupts the usual body boundaries around women and babies – boundaries which extend the individualism which is dominant in the global North to include breast milk – only the birth mother's milk is generally viewed as suitable and appropriate for her baby, unless of course the choice is made to use manufactured formula, or milk from a breast milk bank is 'medically' indicated. The research undertaken by the authors provides data to show how women can work collectively to provide peer milk, as opposed to more formal institutionalized arrangements, to the benefit of both mothers and babies. The in-depth ethnographic approach enables the reader to really understand, not only the reasons behind peer milk sharing, and its utility, but also the social relations and practices which develop through the process. The authors argue that 'peer milk-sharing communities can be conceptualized as bio-communities of practice where bio-intimacy is created through the exchange of biological material and the establishing of (bio-) intimacy and affective bonds between donors and recipients'. They draw on the concept of 'biological citizenship' developed by Nikolas Rose and Carlos Novas, linking this to 'communities of practice' through the process of collectivizing individual biological experiences through activism. They go on to argue that while biological citizenship can help us to understand the relationship between the emergence of community and the biological nature of lactation and infant feeding, it is not sufficient. They utilize Ken Plummer's ideas about intimate citizenship in order to account for the ways in which the practice of milk sharing violates traditional views of bodily boundedness. They go further however, in attempting to show how the materiality of human milk and the labour involved in its production actually affects the particular communities that emerge through milk sharing via networks of 'bio-intimacy'. From there they develop a materialist analysis drawing on the work of Susan Falls and Rhonda Shaw to introduce the concept of 'emotional materiality' linking gifted milk to bio-intimacy as the basis of bio-communities of practice.

The discussion in the book offers a good example of the tensions between expert systems and communal and local arrangements with breast milk banks presented by health professionals, and the media, as safe and peer milk sharing as risky – mothers are not seen as knowing best. The book seeks to 'bridge the gap of understanding' by showing how these different positions have emerged and are located in such a way as to produce mis-information in relation to peer milk sharing. The book provides not only a very interesting account of the social context of milk sharing but an evidence base from which better-informed policy and practice may hopefully emerge to the benefit of women and their babies.

Sue Scott and Stevi Jackson
August 2020

1

Introduction: Sharing Milk

In a time where breastfeeding has re-emerged as the most widely promoted method of infant feeding, a distinct form of sharing breastmilk has emerged in the United States (US) and other post-industrialized societies in the Global North. Parents and other caretakers who are unable to provide sufficient breastmilk themselves are increasingly turning to peers to acquire human milk for their babies. They meet these peers through a combination of online and offline social networks, and form communities with distinct spoken and unspoken rules about how milk sharing takes place. These communities are reflective of emerging socialities made possible by 21st-century advances in technology, new forms of communication, and changing understandings of the human body and its products.

This is a book that analyzes human milk-sharing communities in a large metropolitan area in southeastern US. We have engaged with milk-sharing communities for several years, at times becoming part of them, in our endeavour to understand how these practices are reflective of new and changing ways of establishing and maintaining social connectedness. We describe the practices of milk sharing, the meanings ascribed to human milk, and the labour involved in its production. We build on existing scholarship and theoretical frameworks to develop a model for understanding contemporary forms of bodily sharing.

The feeding of human milk to socially and biologically unrelated infants is not, by any means, a new phenomenon. Rather, it is a normal method of infant feeding documented throughout human history, in societies around the world, and across mammalian species. Nevertheless, Euroamerican values of individualism, the heteropatriarchal nuclear family, and dominant gender roles have generated expectations that mothers throughout the Global North – particularly those who are white, middle-class, heterosexual and cisgender – are individually responsible for feeding their own, and only their own, infants (Shaw

2007, 2015, 2019; Carroll 2014; Palmquist 2015; Falls 2017; Shaw and Morgan 2017; Wilson 2018). This mandate emerges within a broader set of expectations that Sharon Hays (1996) calls 'intensive mothering', in which mothers are expected to maintain individual responsibility for their children's health and wellbeing, consult and follow expert guidance on parenting matters, expend vast time and resources into parenting, and prioritize their children's needs above their own. The widely publicized 'breast is best' mantra mandates that 'good mothers' put forth extensive effort to feed their babies their own exclusive breastmilk (Lee 2007, 2008; Marshall et al 2007; Crossley 2009; Knaak 2010). However, institutional barriers such as lack of paid maternity leave, hospital practices that disrupt breastfeeding, and aggressive formula marketing along with physical discomfort commonly associated with early breastfeeding undermine many mothers' attempts to breastfeed (Van Esterik 1989; Kelleher 2006; Rosenberg et al 2008; Stearns 2009; Tomori et al 2016, 2018). Consequently, although more than 83% of US mothers initiate breastfeeding, only 24.9% meet the American Academy of Pediatrics' (AAP) (2012) recommendation to breastfeed exclusively for the first six months of life (CDC 2018). While most turn to artificial infant formula, a growing number obtain milk from their peers.

In this book, we provide an in-depth, ethnographic analysis of peer breastmilk sharing in Central Florida. We provide detailed accounts of the multiple and varied forms of peer milk sharing that take place in the communities we studied. Dominant discourses often dichotomize two forms of milk sharing that are understood to take place in societies throughout the Global North: the biomedical distribution of processed human milk through milk banks, and peer milk sharing facilitated over the internet through well-known websites such as Eats on Feets and Human Milk 4 Human Babies. In dominant discourses, milk banking is represented as a formalized, institutionally mediated method of procuring and distributing human milk in ways that are lifesaving to medically fragile, premature infants (Carter et al 2015; Carter and Reyes-Foster 2016). Those involved in the practice – breastmilk donors, health professionals, recipient caregivers – are presented as moral subjects, acting only in the best interests of the recipient babies (Carroll 2015; Shaw 2015; Shaw and Morgan 2017). In contrast, peer milk sharing is portrayed as an unregulated activity, contradicting the recommendations of healthcare organizations and professionals. Individuals who participate in milk sharing – parents who donate, and those who receive peer milk – are portrayed as sometimes well intentioned, but ultimately naïve, reckless and immoral (Carter et al

2015; Carter and Reyes-Foster 2016). In dominant discourses, these practices are represented as the primary forms that milk sharing takes in the Global North.

Social science scholarship on milk-sharing practices has proliferated in recent years, which has nuanced this dichotomy between milk banking and online peer milk sharing. Scholars demonstrate that, rather than being a wholly scientific process, milk banking is a social practice whereby human milk is constructed as safe through standardized procedures, scientific processing, and interactional dialogue between physicians and their patients (Shaw 2010; Zizzo 2011; Landers and Hartmann 2013; Carroll 2014, 2015; Carroll et al 2014; Shaw and Morgan 2017). This scholarship also corrects stereotypical ideas about the perceptions, motivations and practices of parents who use well-known websites to share milk, and illuminates other forms that milk sharing takes in contemporary post-industrial societies (Long 2003; Shaw 2007, 2019; Thorley 2009, 2012; Akre et al 2011; Cassidy 2012a, 2012b; Gribble 2013, 2014a, 2014b, 2014c, 2018; Palmquist and Doehler 2014, 2016; Perrin et al 2014; Palmquist 2015; Reyes-Foster et al 2015, 2017; Falls 2017; Carter et al 2018; Cassar-Uhl and Liberatos 2018; Reyes-Foster and Carter 2018a, 2018b; Wilson 2018).

In this book, we contribute to this nuanced understanding of peer milk sharing by illustrating the multiple and varied milk-sharing practices we observed throughout our in-depth, ethnographic investigation. We show how milk banking and peer milk sharing via the internet represent two ends of a spectrum of milk-sharing practices that occur with varied degrees of intervention and encouragement from healthcare professionals. As the stories we report throughout the book illuminate, peer milk sharing unfolds in a variety of ways in contemporary societies in the Global North. Thus, our research builds on expanded definitions of *what* constitutes peer milk sharing, and our analysis deepens social scientific understanding of how and why parents and other caregivers engage in the practice.

In addition to illustrating the varied practices that constitute peer milk sharing, we also analyze *how* it takes place. We describe the individual practices of donors and recipients, the dyadic relationships between them, and the broader collective of individuals who form milk sharing communities. We build on existing scholarship on the communities and relationships that constitute and are constituted by peer breastmilk sharing (Cassidy 2012a, 2012b; Perrin et al 2014; Palmquist 2015; Falls 2017; Gribble 2018; Wilson 2018), and add to this literature a conceptualization of peer milk-sharing communities as 'bio-communities of practice'. Our concept of bio-communities of practice, further developed in Chapter 2, combines insights regarding the organizational structure of informal communities from Wenger and colleagues' (Lave 1991; Lave and Wenger 1991; Wenger 1999, 2010; Wenger and Snyder 2000) concept of 'communities of practice', with theories of reproductive belonging and connectedness through 'bio-intimacy' (Shaw and Morgan 2017; Shaw 2019) and 'bio-citizenship' (Rose and Novas 2005; Halse 2009, 2012). Conceptualizing milk sharers as communities of practice highlights the goal-oriented nature of their actions. Expanding this concept facilitates understanding of the social and biological connections between individuals who participate in the practice.

Discovering milk sharing

It was a sunny Tuesday morning in Central Florida when I (Shannon) arrived at Jane's ranch-style home in a small city just outside of Orlando. It had been about a year since Jane and I had last seen each other, though we kept in touch over Facebook. We hugged, chatted briefly about how our morning was going so far, talked about how much her daughters had grown since I had seen them last, and sat down in her cosy family room to talk about milk sharing. While we talked, Jane's six-year-old daughter, Avery, happily played with their chocolate Labrador before completing her maths home-schooling work, and Jane attended to her youngest daughter, Sadie, breastfeeding her as needed throughout the interview. As I sat comfortably on Jane's couch and she rocked in her recliner, she recounted her milk-sharing experience.

Jane had always had an abundance of milk, and initially began expressing it after Avery's birth to provide comfort and avoid having her breasts become engorged and painful with too much milk. A stay-at-home mother at the time, Jane spent most of her time at home with Avery, having no use for the expressed milk. After about four months, she found her freezer filling up. She wasn't sure what to do with the milk, as she knew her daughter didn't need it, but it seemed too precious to throw out. She attended a breastfeeding group at Mother's Love Birth Center, where we both had given birth, mostly as a way of meeting other mothers; it was at this group that Jane and I first met. I remembered the incident as Jane recounted how she – and also how I – was first introduced to peer milk sharing in early December of 2009:

> 'I had oversupply with my first daughter so I was only pumping to be comfortable, but I had too much milk and I couldn't figure out what to do with it. So, I went to a

> breastfeeding support group and pretty much asked, "What do I do with this?" And I was lucky because that day there was actually a mom there that was looking for donor milk. So, right when the group finished, we went straight over to the midwife and I got a blood test per her request that she paid for and I started donating my milk to her. And I donated my milk to her exclusively for six months and was able to keep her baby off of formula because of it. So that's how I got started, I pretty much just asked because I didn't know what to do with all the extra milk.'

As Jane recounted her entry into peer milk sharing, I remembered the incident vividly. Jane and I had met only a few weeks earlier as members of the breastfeeding support group that had just started after the reopening of Mother's Love Birth Center at its new location. I remember Kendall, Jane's first breastmilk recipient, walking into the meeting holding her two-week-old baby, sitting down cross-legged on the floor, and bursting into tears as she told the story of her daily paediatrician visits, her daughter Amelia's declining weight, her suspicion that she wasn't producing enough breastmilk for her, Amelia's recent diagnosis as failing to thrive, and her doctor's assertion that she would have to switch to formula if Amelia didn't gain weight by the end of the week. With tears streaming down her face, Kendall told us how committed she was to breastfeeding, how hard she had tried, and how she felt devastated and betrayed by her body for not being able to provide enough milk to feed baby Amelia. I remember Jane saying to her quietly, "I have extra milk that I'm not using if you want it."

Although Jane began peer milk sharing as a way of managing extra milk, she wound up implementing a routine that would allow her to express milk every day for the next six months for baby Amelia. Now on her second child, Jane estimates that she has shared "a couple thousand" ounces of milk with a dozen or so recipients, pumping and donating about a hundred ounces each week. A birth doula and Certified Lactation Counsellor (CLC)[1] herself – training she received after Avery was no longer an infant but before she was pregnant with Sadie – Jane is well educated on the properties of breastmilk, proper handling and storage techniques, and common breastfeeding issues and problems. She believes strongly that breastmilk provides benefits to babies that are unparalleled by infant formula and empathizes with mothers who are unable to provide their own breastmilk to their babies. She believes peer-shared breastmilk is far healthier than infant formula, stating, "I don't think you can have an opinion on it because it's science.

Human breastmilk, no matter how it's given, is preferable to formula." Jane is well known among many local maternity care providers and is integrated in several local mothering communities. She typically finds breastmilk recipients through birth professionals, friends, and word of mouth, often connected through Facebook, and also donates to the local non-profit milk-sharing organization Get Pumped.[2] Although Jane acknowledges that her family would certainly benefit from extra money, and she is not personally opposed to the purchase and sale of human milk, she feels that her milk is something she can give to others, and because it is unique and temporary and she is able, she chooses to give it for as long as she can. With some recipients, she establishes long-term relationships; other relationships are short-lived, and some recipients she never meets.

Looking back, Jane could not have predicted how her introduction to peer milk sharing would affect the course of the next several years of her life. Neither could Shannon. I (Shannon) come to the current project as a mother of three children (Joshua, Ella and Auguste) who was first exposed to peer breastmilk sharing at the breastfeeding support group at Mother's Love Birth Center in 2009. As I became more involved in the group, I witnessed several mothers around me sharing milk. At times Mother's Love Birth Center would collect milk for a needy baby, and I learned about the local breastmilk-sharing organization Get Pumped. The breastfeeding support group evolved into a non-profit breastfeeding support organization, The Breastfeeding Project, which provided free lactation education and support to local mothers. Over the next decade, I remained active in Central Florida breastfeeding communities through ongoing participation in private and public Facebook groups, community events, and breastfeeding support groups. I witnessed peer breastmilk sharing in the various forms that we report on, including cross-nursing, requesting donations on the internet, sharing among friends, and collection through organizations, midwives and other healthcare providers.

My motivation for this project is to facilitate representations of caregivers who participate in breastmilk sharing that more accurately reflect how and why they engage in the practice than is conveyed by dominant discourses. When considering a new project in 2013 within my broader research area of the sociology of reproduction, I searched for literature on peer breastmilk sharing, finding only a few articles published on the topic at that time. I came across several articles that expressed opposition to milk sharing, but little discussion of what the practice looked like, who was participating in it, and why they were doing it. I wanted to conduct a research project that would portray a more accurate portrait of what peer milk sharing looks like in practice, and why individuals engage in it. Since that time, scholarship on the topic has flourished, and I am grateful to be able to engage in conversation with other social scientists who share a similar passion for accurate representations and detailed analysis of milk sharing.

I come to the project as a mother who was fortunate to have the support, resources and physical capacity to exclusively breastfeed my own children well beyond their first birthdays. As a graduate student with my first child and professor with my second two, I had enough flexibility in my schedule that I was able to work from home on days I was not scheduled to teach, where I would often spend my days breastfeeding and caretaking while writing, responding to student emails, and prepping for classes on my laptop. On days I had to work on campus, I pumped in my private office and during my commute home. I never experienced issues with milk supply, but I also rarely had extra milk in the freezer. There were three occasions when I was asked to donate milk to a friend or friend of a friend, and I was able to donate at least a few bags of milk each time, totalling around 200 ounces. Although I developed relationships with many women in the communities we studied, and I would describe Jane as a friend, most of the mothers I interviewed and observed were unknown to me outside of this research.

Beatriz comes to this project also as a mother of three sons (Aydin, Rowan and Miles) who tried, unsuccessfully, to exclusively breastfeed her three children. With my first child, I (Beatriz) continually struggled to produce enough milk, finally giving up after three months of undergoing stressful weight checks, seeking advice from expensive lactation consultants and other specialists, and trying every supplement on the market. I hoped that the stressful circumstances of my son's birth and his initial stay in a neonatal intensive care unit (NICU) were the reasons for our breastfeeding woes, and I was determined that I would be able to breastfeed my second child. After all, everything I had read about breastfeeding attributed insufficient milk production to lack of societal support. When my first was born, I was a graduate student, subsisting on very little money, facing financial and emotional stress. By the time I was pregnant with my second child, I held a stable, well-paid job and had a supportive environment around me. There was no reason, I believed, that I could not produce enough milk.

When I met Shannon, I was just finishing the first trimester of this second pregnancy. I had just completed a research project on mental health and psychiatry in Mexico, and I was looking for a project that would not take me far from home. I had become interested in the anthropology of reproduction and was introduced to Shannon by our mutual colleague, Amanda Koontz. When Shannon brought up human milk sharing, my initial reaction was surprise. "You can do that?," I thought, immediately thinking of what a difference that might have made in my own life.

When Rowan was born a few months later, under conditions that should have been ideal for supporting breastfeeding, we found ourselves, once again, facing the painful reality of insufficient milk production. He simply wasn't gaining enough weight on the amount of milk I was producing. After months of frustration and tears, my spouse and I finally decided to feed him shared milk at the same time that Shannon and I were conducting participant observation research on milk sharing. A friend of ours, Jill, who was a gestational surrogate, had recently given birth and was donating her milk. She became our primary donor and I continued to breastfeed my child, supplementing with her milk until he was nearly one. After his first birthday, I continued to nurse him until he was three years old. Rowan is the only baby I gave shared milk to, and also the one with whom I had the longest and most satisfying breastfeeding relationship. By the time Miles came along, Shannon and I had transitioned away from ethnographic engagement and, while I again experienced insufficient breastmilk production, I did not have the ability to engage in the extensive labour necessary to secure donor milk. I made the decision to supplement with formula with no regret. While Shannon has the experience of being a milk donor, I have the experience of becoming a recipient. I also bring an intersectional perspective to this work through my position as a woman of colour and as an immigrant who grew up in the US. My background as a cultural outsider in this group – our sample is overwhelmingly white, US-born, and socioeconomically privileged – affords our project a unique vantage point and adds nuance to our analysis.

As feminist scholars, we think all people should have the right to feed their babies how they choose, and we see that there are structural constraints that limit individuals' freedom in this realm. In addition, informed choice requires access to knowledge, and the current lack of information on peer milk sharing makes its safety impossible to fully assess. We hope that by contributing to the gap in knowledge about peer milk sharing, this work can help reduce some of those constraints.

Milk sharing in context

Peer breastmilk sharing, sometimes also referred to as 'peer-to-peer milk sharing' (Gribble 2012, 2013, 2014a, 2014b, 2014c, 2018), 'informal milk sharing' (Palmquist 2015), 'co-feeding' (Thorley 2009, 2012), 'cross-nursing' (Shaw 2007), 'breast sharing' (Long 2003), or 'allomaternal nursing' (Hewlett and Winn 2014), is defined as the non-remunerated transfer of human milk from one caregiver to another for the purpose of feeding a child. Occurring outside of formal institutional or governmental oversight, peer milk sharing is typically arranged by individuals in society. Although peer milk sharing has taken place throughout human history and across many cultures, it has gained attention in the Global North during the past decade due to the creation of two peer milk-sharing organizations in 2010 – Human Milk 4 Human Babies (see Figure 1.1) and Eats on Feets – which each use the internet to facilitate peer breastmilk sharing (Cassidy 2012a). These organizations operate hundreds of Facebook pages throughout the world to assist the local exchange of human milk, facilitating tens of thousands of milk exchanges annually (Gribble 2014a). The organizations do not screen donors or evaluate the milk, but they do recommend that participants engage in safe milk-sharing practices. Eats on Feets recommends that participants abide by the 'four pillars of safe breastmilk sharing', which include informed choice, donor screening, safe milk handling, and home pasteurization (Eats on Feets n.d.). These organizations' use of new technologies – specifically the internet and social media – to facilitate the transfer of human milk has caused alarm among public health policy makers, despite a lack of comprehensive social scientific information about how and why peer milk sharing takes place within local communities. This book contributes to the growing body of literature in this area by providing an in-depth exploration of peer milk-sharing practices within a single geographic location.

A global history of milk sharing

The notion that an infant should be fed its mother's – and *only* its mother's – own milk is consistent with Euroamerican cultural logic, premised on a belief that human beings are self-contained, rational individuals who act in their own best interests (Shaw 2007, 2015, 2019; Falls 2017; Shaw and Morgan 2017; Lee 2018a; Wilson 2018). This construct, often referred to as the 'neoliberal subject' (Rose 1996), engages in a continual effort to surveil and care for its own self, a process referred to as 'governmentality', the mindset of governing the self, releasing the state from its obligation while maintaining its prerogative to sustain and manage life (Foucault 1978, 2003). Neoliberal subjects are rational, self-interested and self-actualizing. They can be

Figure 1.1: Human Milk 4 Human Babies meme

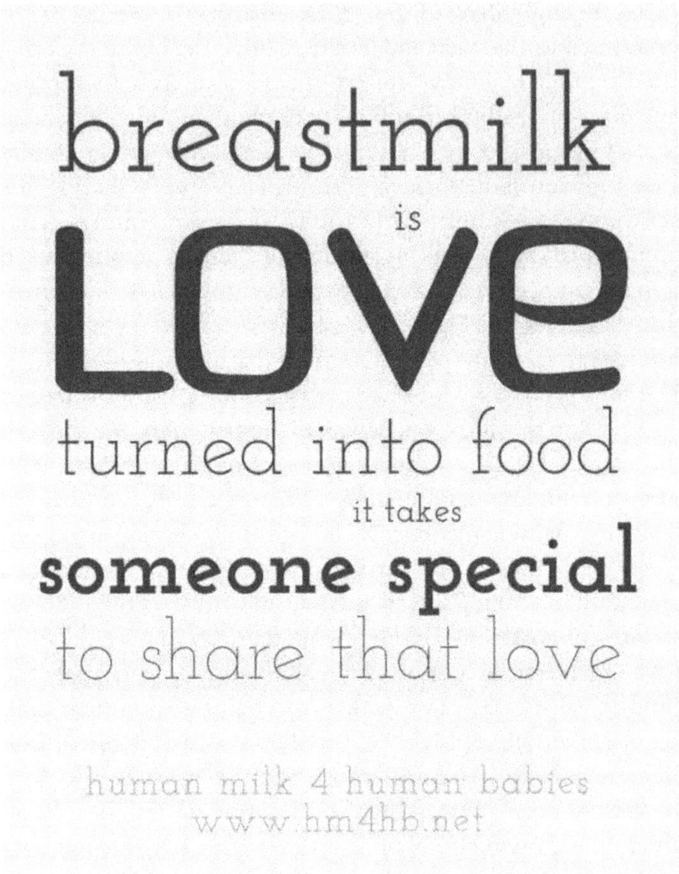

Source: Courtesy of Human Milk 4 Human Babies

trusted to act in their own self-interest, which in turn happens to align with the self-interest of the state. Governmentality allows neoliberal subjects to internalize state priorities to sustain and manage life. Based on this construct, contemporary understandings of 'intensive mothering' (Hays 1996) depart from this *a priori* understanding of human behaviour: mothers will (and should) prioritize their own children above the children of others.

We can appreciate the limits of the construct of the neoliberal subject in the ethnographic record, particularly when it comes to infant feeding. Across the world, we see that nursing mothers can and frequently do feed infants who are not their biological children (Van Esterik 2002; Long 2003; Thorley 2009, 2012; Hewlett and Winn 2014). This practice is estimated to occur in more than 90%

of cultures, though it falls outside the norm in most (Hewlett and Winn 2014). Co-feeding is particularly common in societies where cooperation is integral to the survival of the group (Van Esterik 2002). It is common in many hunter and gatherer societies, especially those living in tropical forest environments. However, environmental factors alone do not determine co-feeding practices, as they are also shaped by cultural norms. For example, co-feeding is normative within the Aka culture but strictly prohibited among the Ngandu, both hunter and gatherer societies who share similar natural environments (Hewlett and Winn 2014).

Beyond hunter and gatherer societies, co-feeding is most commonly observed in cultures in the Middle East, Central America and the Caribbean, and Oceania, followed by Africa and Asia, and less commonly observed in Europe and North and South America (Hewlett and Winn 2014). In most societies, co-feeding is practised in emergency situations, especially maternal death, illness, or inability to produce milk. Only a few societies have such strong prohibitions against co-feeding that an infant would presumably die without their own mother's milk. In societies where co-feeding is common or permitted, including hunter and gatherer societies, it is typically a close relative, especially a grandmother, who breastfeeds a young infant, usually ending by the time the infant is 12 months of age even when breastfeeding continues to age two or three (Hewlett and Winn 2014). Co-feeding is also common in some non-industrial societies across the world that believe that colostrum – the thick, nutrient-dense substance typically produced in the first few days before the milk comes in – is dangerous to infant health. These societies often have taboos against maternal breastfeeding in the first few days, and instead a grandmother, midwife, or other relative will breastfeed the infant until the mother's colostrum is replaced by milk (Lozoff 1983; Hewlett and Winn 2014).

Some societies where co-feeding is common, particularly in the Middle East, practise 'milk kinship', where kinship ties are created through the consumption of breastmilk (Altorki 1980; Carsten 1995; Parkes 2004). Most often, the infant who receives breastmilk becomes part of the donating mother's kin group. Non-biological children maintain ties with their 'milk mothers' and may feel obligated to provide for them in older age (Cassidy and El Tom 2010; Ramli and Ibrahim 2010). Relationships among 'milk siblings' – unrelated children who have consumed milk from the same mother – are regulated by beliefs that their offspring would be 'deformed' if they reproduced together. Although the concept of milk kinship predates Islam, rules prohibiting marriage between milk siblings are formalized in Islamic family law (Long 2003). In the Hindu Kush of Northern Pakistan, milk kinship was used as a strategy to foster community exogamy and create alliances (Parkes 2001).

Wet nursing, defined as the nursing of a child by a woman who is compensated or coerced to do so (Shaw 2007), was commonplace in European history (Fildes 1987; Golden 1996) as well as other socially stratified Eurasian societies including Korea and Malaysia, and among African kingdoms such as the Ashanti and Buganda (Hewlett and Winn 2014). Whereas co-feeding strengthens social bonds within a group, the historiography of wet nursing suggests that this practice was generally exploitative, frequently resulting in the death of the wet nurses' own infants (Shaw 2007). Wet nurses were treated with suspicion by their employers, who saw them as socially inferior beings prone to unpredictable and immoral impulses (Wolf 1999). Wet nurses particularly those who were unmarried, were suspected of being vectors for venereal disease, yet they were much more vulnerable to contracting illnesses from their charges. This is particularly true in the case of syphilis, which is difficult to transmit from wet nurse to infant but which has a nearly 100% rate of transmission from infant to wet nurse (Kertzer 1999). Wet nurses were exploited in other ways as well: for example, in the 18th century, they were used in early experimental treatment of syphilis, where they were exposed to large amounts of mercury, a highly toxic heavy metal, in hopes that their mercury-infected milk could treat their charges' congenital syphilis (Sherwood 1995). This exploitation of wet nurses is crystalized in the practice of forcing Black enslaved women to nurse their owners' infants, frequently at the expense of their own children, in the US antebellum south (Blum 1999; A Negro Nurse 2001; Shaw 2007; Harrison 2016).

The invention of the electric breast pump disconnected breastmilk from women's bodies, who no longer had to put nurslings to the breast in order to nourish them (Bar-Yam 2010). At the same time, a gradual shift began taking place away from professional wet nursing towards uncompensated milk donation (Swanson 2014). While 20th-century physicians believed that breastmilk was the perfect food for infants and that access to breastmilk could make the difference between life and death, they recognized that hiring a wet nurse could bring significant challenges for caregivers (Golden 1996). Consistent with the development of scientific medicine, the need to measure and pasteurize donor milk led to the creation of the first Mother's Breastmilk stations (Swanson 2011). Rather than breastfeed needy babies directly, wet nurses would express their milk under medical supervision at the stations, where they would receive payment by the ounce (Swanson 2011). The milk was then blended, pasteurized, bottled and dispensed. This shift away from wet nursing towards the use of expressed milk coincided with growing ambivalence towards wet nursing from mothers (Wolf 1999). During the 1960s and 1970s, hospital-based Mother's Milk stations gave way to milk banks, which at the time were run more like 'swaps of outgrown clothes and baby toys' (Swanson 2011: 754).

Importantly, milk exchanged from these early banks was freely given, not sold (Swanson 2011). This reverse commodification – from paid wet nursing to free donation – was eventually formalized, in the US, into the code of ethics of the Human Milk Banking Association of North America (HMBANA). Meanwhile, the discovery of pasteurization and hygienic innovations informed by germ theory resulted in the creation of safe and inexpensive alternatives to human milk, most notably infant formula (Law 2000). In her study of wet nurses in Chicago in the early 20th century, Jacqueline Wolf (1999) concludes that ambivalence towards wet nurses, combined with the innovation of infant formula and the emergence of bottle feeding, led to the eventual disappearance of the practice and contributed to the definitive shift from breast to bottle feeding. Meanwhile, as Swanson documents, early milk 'banks', stored in women's freezers and freely gifted, gave way to formal milk banking in the 1980s. In response to the AIDS crisis, and increased understanding of the potential to transmit HIV through breastmilk, HMBANA was established in 1985 to create industry standards for the collection, testing, homogenization and pasteurization of donor milk (Bar-Yam 2010; Swanson 2014).

Today, there are 28 HMBANA-affiliated milk banks in the US and Canada and several more that are developing (HMBANAa n.d.). Milk banks collect breastmilk from donors who have been screened for health and lifestyle practices, medications and illnesses, and have had their blood tested for infectious diseases (Bar-Yam 2010; Carroll 2014). The banks pasteurize donated milk to eliminate pathogens and distribute the processed milk to needy infants, including those born prematurely and receiving care in NICUs (Updegrove 2013). Banked human milk is distributed based on physician prescription and therefore is not available for many parents who wish to feed their healthy babies human milk over formula. Although HMBANA milk banks are non-profit organizations and breastmilk donors are not compensated for their milk, these protocols cost money, which is factored into the price of donated milk (Carroll and Herrmann 2013), a cost that is usually passed on to hospitals and sometimes to public and private health insurance companies. The average cost of banked milk is US$4 per ounce (Carroll and Herrmann 2013). Currently, six states (New York, California, Missouri, Kansas, Texas and Utah) provide Medicaid coverage for donor milk. As milk banks have proliferated, so have for-profit, bioventure capitalist companies looking to find ways to make breastmilk lucrative.

Human milk in the capitalist market

'In an era when the benefits of breast milk are better understood and more scientifically certain than ever, demand for it has created a niche industry,' reads a *Wired* magazine byline to a story about the market for breast milk (Dutton 2011). The 2010s have seen a slew of similar publications focused on the ways breastmilk, valued as 'liquid gold', has become a hot commodity. Many of these articles focus on the two most visible corporate players in the world of breastmilk capitalism: the for-profit corporations Medolac Laboratories and Prolacta Bioscience. Medolac advertises shelf-stable 'commercially-sterile human milk products for use in the hospital or at home' (Medolac 2018) while Prolacta calls itself 'the pioneer in standardized human milk-based nutritional products for premature infants in the neonatal intensive care unit (NICU)' (Prolacta 2018). Functioning much like pharmaceutical companies, Medolac and Prolacta have created human milk-based products marketed to hospitals and parents seeking human milk for their infants.

The new societal valuing of human milk has resulted in three different forms of milk transfer: two 'markets'[3] and one gift economy. The first market for human milk does not involve direct consumers, but rather involves bio-capitalist companies and non-profit human milk banks vying for hospital NICUs to purchase their processed human milk. This market is self-regulated, conforming to standards and best practices agreed, for better or worse, by all parties (Bar-Yam 2010; Hassan 2010; Swanson 2014). The second market is a 'grey' market, an unregulated, informal marketplace (Fomaro 2003; Bowman 2008; Totenberg 2013) where individuals sell their unprocessed milk directly to buyers, often using the internet to find each other. The milk-classifieds website Only The Breast is one such venue that facilitates this market, but Craigslist, despite prohibiting the sale of human milk on its platform, is also known to be used for this purpose. Finally, the milk-sharing gift economy is the one where most of our work is located: the usually community-based, free exchange of human milk. Within the gift economy of milk sharing, small tokens of appreciation, such as gift cards or milk storage bags, and other forms of reciprocity are considered appropriate, but the outright exchange of money is not (Gribble 2013, 2018; Shaw 2007, 2015, 2019; Falls 2017). In this section, we briefly explore each of these sites of exchange, elucidating how human milk both assumes and resists commodification.

For-profit companies Medolac Laboratories and Prolacta Bioscience comprise part of 'bio-capitalism', corporations that, through research and development, seek to bring new biological technologies into the capitalist market (Peters and Venkatesan 2010). This includes the manufacture and sale of products derived from human biological material, including organs, tissues, cells, blood, embryos, semen and milk (Waldby and Mitchell 2006; Twine 2017). This human biological material, seen as 'hazardous' or 'waste' in other contexts, is imbued with what Catherine Waldby and Robert Mitchell (Waldby and Mitchell 2006) identify as 'biovalue' by undergoing a technological transformation in the manufacturing process. Medolac produces a shelf-stable, commercially sterile human milk that it sells to hospitals at a cost of US$5.75 per ounce, slightly higher than the US$4 per ounce charged for pasteurized donor milk by HMBANA-affiliated human milk banks. Meanwhile, Prolacta Bioscience produces a 'human milk fortifier' made from human milk and sold to hospital nurseries at US$184 per ounce (Fentiman 2009). Medolac's and Prolacta's products are marketed as 'scientific', 'sterile' and 'safe', whereas human milk in other settings is frequently portrayed as unhygienic and dangerous (Carter et al 2015; Carter and Reyes-Foster 2016). This contrast can at times extend to processed human milk from non-profit HMBANA-affiliated milk banks, as Medolac marketed its shelf-stable milk as the 'only commercially sterile' human milk product available, safer even than the pasteurized donor milk available from milk banks.

Meanwhile, while presenting itself as a public benefit organization, the bioventure capitalist company Medolac's prime competition happens to be HMBANA milk banks. Perhaps recognizing that most consumers on the ground are unwilling to treat human milk as a commodity, or unable to pay nearly US$6 per ounce, Medolac's primary goal is to sell its product to hospitals, supplanting HMBANA milk banks as a provider of donor milk to vulnerable infants.

HMBANA has long advocated for the non-profit availability of human milk to the most vulnerable infants. In its own position statement on the ethical allocation of human milk, HMBANA states, 'HMBANA does not endorse the practice of selling or purchasing human milk, human milk components, or human milk by-products', noting that commodification places undue pressure on mothers to become donors at the expense of their own infant's needs (HMBNAb n.d.). The statement continues as follows:

> Women donate to non-profit banks for altruistic reasons rather than for personal gain … [HMBANA] does not condone, and in fact, questions the practice of buying and selling milk as a commodity. Introducing the profit motive could put the infant of the lactating mother at risk if she feels pressure to provide a certain volume of milk to a bank or a recipient rather than feeding her own infant. (HMBANAb n.d.)

The notion that human milk sharing, be it in the form of direct peer sharing or through an organization such as a milk bank, should be non-profit has found societal echo. Recognizing this, bioventure capitalist companies continue to represent themselves to a broader audience with the implication that human milk should be kept separate from profit motives (Hassan 2010). In 2018, Medolac's website, for instance, featured prominent messaging such as 'more than profit', placing its status as a public benefit corporation (a specific type of corporation that lists public benefit in its charter but remains profit-driven) front and centre, noting: 'As a public benefit company, our decisions are driven by what's best for babies, not solely the bottom line. We can make decisions that other companies, beholden to investors or stockholders, can't' (Medolac 2018). Medolac's milk-collecting arm, the Mothers Milk Cooperative, presents itself as a non-profit, cooperatively owned milk bank, despite the fact that donated milk is only used to produce Medolac's shelf-stable milk and that Medolac founder Elena Medo sits on its board of directors. It is through the Mothers Milk Cooperative that donors may be compensated up to one dollar per ounce for their milk. Likewise, Medolac competitor Prolacta also collects milk through non-HMBANA milk banks that also compensate their donors one dollar per ounce. Prolacta also presents itself as a benevolent force: as early as 2009, the company encouraged women to donate their milk to HIV-positive babies in Africa. They then sent only 25% of the donated milk to Africa, and used the remaining 75% to manufacture their human milk-based fortifier and sell it to US hospitals (Fentiman 2009).

Medolac's and Prolacta's deliberate downplaying of their profit motive is reflective of societal attitudes towards the commodification of human milk. Within milk-sharing circles, commodification is seen as taboo, frequently rejected as immoral and suspect. Among our study participants as well as those studied by other social scientists

(Shaw 2007, 2015, 2019; Gribble 2013, 2014a, 2014b; Palmquist 2015; Palmquist and Doehler 2016; Falls 2017; Wilson 2018), peer milk sharing takes place within a gift economy, one in which compensation is neither expected nor desired. In her analysis of milk sharing in a metropolitan area of the US South, Falls argues that the rejection of commodification of milk is a rejection 'of the reduction of life to capital ... a resistance to bio-capitalism' (2017: 165). The gift of milk is thus laden with social significance. While our research participants were also resistant to the commodification of milk, we found their responses were laden with a complex view of the morality of selling and its connection to motherhood and the human reproductive body.

Perspectives on milk sharing

In 2010, the creation of online peer milk sharing organizations Eats on Feets and Human Milk 4 Human Babies brought public attention to milk sharing in the Global North, seemingly premised on the notion that the organizations had rejuvenated an outdated practice that had been all but eliminated (Akre et al 2011; Cassidy 2012a). Several healthcare clinicians and researchers published critiques of milk sharing, presenting it as a newly re-emerging practice, and using risk-based language to highlight the associated 'dangers'. An article in the *American Journal of Nursing* (Nelson 2012) is titled "Breast Milk Sharing is Making a Comeback, But Should It?", followed by the abstract "Internet access provides convenience but carries real risk." Many of the critiques conflate breastmilk sharing with breastmilk selling (for example, Geraghty et al 2011, 2013; Nelson 2012; Steele et al 2015), warning that sellers could increase the volume of milk by adding cow's milk or other substances to boost their profits, and emphasizing the potential spread of infectious disease or illness from environmental contamination, poor hygiene, or substance use among donors or sellers. Other critiques came from a legal standpoint, highlighting a lack of government oversight, and urging federal and state lawmakers to 'consider adopting specific regulations governing the sale, processing, and shipment of human milk, particularly with regard to impersonal and informal internet sales, to better ensure the health and safety of children in these potentially dangerous transactions' (David 2011: 166). Beyond notions of risk, other critics argued that peer milk sharing decreases the availability of processed human milk by encouraging peer sharing rather than donation to milk banks, and that it undermines breastfeeding by providing an alternative to adequate breastfeeding resources and support for mothers who experience breastfeeding difficulties or insufficient milk supply (Jones 2013).

Some healthcare experts have critiqued these views, instead calling for research and resources to make peer milk sharing as safe as possible. Karleen Gribble and Bernice L. Hausman (2012) point out that all forms of infant feeding carry some degree of risk, and that public health officials provide recommendations for minimizing risks related to breastfeeding and infant formula feeding. They argue that the prohibitionist stance against peer milk sharing reflects a cultural distaste for sharing breastmilk – what Rhonda Shaw (2004) calls the 'yuk factor' – rather than research-based recommendations. They examine each risk associated with milk sharing, identifying comparable risks with other forms of infant feeding, along with methods for minimizing risks in peer-shared milk, and conclude that health agencies should publicize risk management guidelines rather than proscribing peer milk sharing altogether. James Akre and colleagues (2011) argue that safe models of peer milk sharing could expand the global supply of human milk, thereby improving infant health worldwide, and encourage critics to examine the biases driving their rejection of the practice. They argue that opposition to peer milk sharing is a contemporary manifestation of longstanding suspicion toward women's reproductive bodies, based on views that negative characteristics and bad morals can be passed to children through breastmilk. Further, they argue that peer milk sharing, especially methods that use the internet, are interpreted as challenging the medical establishment, as it takes place outside of medical control. They also question whether peer milk sharing actually threatens donations to milk banks, as many who wish to donate are turned away, a point reinforced in later research (Cassidy 2012a; Gribble 2013, 2014b; Perrin et al 2016).

In mainstream media, peer milk sharing is portrayed in conflicting and contradictory ways, but largely characterized as a dangerous and risky practice. Newspaper articles portray peer milk donors as potentially altruistic yet having questionable morals, and caregivers who receive peer milk as naïve and misinformed, recklessly putting their children in harm's way by feeding them peer breastmilk (Carter et al 2015). The milk itself is cast as risky and dangerous, and its use for infant feeding likened in one widely used quote to 'playing a game of Russian roulette with your baby'. Articles utilize statements from health professionals who oppose milk sharing as 'expert testimonies' and they imagine 'hypothetical atrocities' that *could* – but never *have* – happened that threaten the lives of innocent babies as a result of using peer-shared milk (Carter and Reyes-Foster 2016). These messages educate the public about new forms of milk sharing taking shape on the internet, but they portray them as risky and irresponsible.

Public health organizations have also responded to the development of internet-facilitated peer milk sharing. In the same year that Human Milk 4 Human Babies and Eats on Feets launched, the US Food and Drug Administration (FDA) (USFDA 2010) released a statement warning parents against the use of peer-shared milk. Public health agencies in France and Canada released similar statements (Gribble and Hausman 2012). The FDA's statement includes, in bold and italicized font, 'FDA recommends against feeding your baby breast milk acquired directly from individuals or through the internet' (USFDA 2010). Similarly, the AAP (2012, 2017) included a statement against peer breastmilk sharing in its 2012 and 2017 policy statements on breastfeeding and the use of human milk and donor human milk for the high-risk infant. These official statements were disseminated without any scientific evidence regarding the safety of peer-shared breastmilk or social scientific knowledge of how and why parents engage in the practice (Gribble and Hausman 2012).

In 2016, the American Academy of Nursing (AAN) (2016) released a statement that broke from the prohibitionist stance of other health agencies and institutions. The AAN statement said that some parents will choose to participate in peer breastmilk sharing, and therefore recommended that practitioners discuss the relative risks and benefits with their patients, and educate them on methods for reducing risks, including donor screening and flash heating. International organizations have also taken more nuanced positions. The Academy of Breastfeeding Medicine (ABM) (Sriraman et al 2018) released a position statement in 2018 recommending that healthcare providers educate patients on risk-management strategies for informal milk sharing, particularly donor screening and safe milk-handling practices. Similarly, the World Health Organization (WHO), in its *Global Strategy on Infant and Young Child Feeding* (WHO 2002), suggests a healthy wet nurse as a viable option when a mother's own milk is not available.

Similar to early critiques of peer milk sharing and official statements against it, early biomedical research on breastmilk sharing conflated milk sharing and milk selling. A team of researchers conducted a series of analyses of breastmilk purchased anonymously online and found high levels of bacteria, evidence of cow's milk adulteration, and traces of nicotine in their sample (Keim et al 2013, 2015; Geraghty et al 2015). Subsequent social scientific research (Gribble 2014a, 2014b; Palmquist and Doehler 2014; Reyes-Foster et al 2015; Falls 2017; Wilson 2018) problematized the conflation of milk sharing with milk selling, and newer biomedical research has been conducted that more accurately reflects peer milk-sharing practices. This research, while in its early stages, has thus far found no evidence that shared milk contains higher levels of potentially harmful bacteria than mothers' own milk (Perrin et al 2018).

Milk sharing in practice

Peer milk sharing today

Despite social commentary portraying peer milk sharing as non-existent in the Global North during the late 20th and early 21st centuries, limited existing research suggests otherwise. Virginia Thorley (2009) documents forms of peer milk sharing that took place in Australia from 1978–2008 among mothers who were committed to feeding exclusive breastmilk to their children during times that they were absent or temporarily unable to provide their own milk. Thorley (2012) also documents cases of breastmilk sharing highlighted in western media outlets, such as after a natural disaster or the death of a mother. Similarly, Debbi Long (2003) identified several circumstances that prompted milk sharing among mothers who gave birth in an urban Australian hospital between October 1999 and September 2000, including maternal or infant illness, supplementing a mother's milk supply, or breastfeeding while providing childcare. Rhonda Shaw (2007) describes a highly publicized incident in New Zealand in 1996 whereby a mother became upset that another mother breastfed her crying baby in her absence, highlighting the significance of consent in milk sharing. In our survey, several mothers in the US reported sharing milk in the 1980s and 1990s. This scholarship shows that peer milk sharing continued to be practised in the Global North in recent times, though largely occurring privately or in exceptional circumstances.

In the decade following the creation of Eats on Feets and Human Milk 4 Human Babies, social scientific research has provided a clearer understanding of breastmilk sharing in societies in the Global North, including the US. A national survey (O'Sullivan et al 2018) of 429 US mothers was conducted to assess the prevalence of milk sharing, finding that nearly all participants (94%) had heard of infants being fed another mother's breastmilk. Among survey participants, 17% reported ever participating in some form of human milk sharing, with 12% giving and 6.8% receiving breastmilk. Another survey of 475 breastfeeding mothers who reported having low milk supply found that almost one third (29.1%) reported using peer-shared milk to meet at least 10% of their infants' milk needs (Cassar-Uhl and Liberatos 2018). Although the surveys are not nationally representative, they suggest that peer milk sharing is more common than many people might assume.

Social scientists have identified patterns among people who participate in peer milk sharing. Breastmilk sharing recipients are caregivers of infants or young children who are committed to feeding breastmilk, but who are unable to provide it themselves. Most milk-sharing recipients tend to be mothers who breastfeed their babies, but experience difficulties producing enough milk to exclusively breastfeed and therefore use peer milk to supplement their own breastmilk (Palmquist and Doehler 2014 , 2016; Reyes-Foster et al 2015; Falls 2017; Cassar-Uhl and Liberatos 2018). Parents who are transgender, or those who become parents though surrogacy, foster care or adoption, may also become peer milk recipients, and peer milk may also be used in cases of maternal death (Palmquist and Doehler 2014; MacDonald et al 2016; Falls 2017; Giles 2017; Wilson 2018). In the US, parents who share milk are disproportionately white, college-educated and socioeconomically privileged, and peer-shared milk is most commonly fed to healthy, full-term babies (Palmquist and Doehler 2014, 2016; Reyes-Foster et al 2015; Cassar-Uhl and Liberatos 2018). Peer milk donors are typically mothers who are breastfeeding and produce more milk than their own children consume (Gribble 2014b; Palmquist and Doehler 2014, 2016; Palmquist 2015; Reyes-Foster et al 2015). Individuals who serve as surrogates may also express milk after birth to give to the surrogate parents, to a milk bank, or to peers (Carroll 2015; Palmquist and Doehler 2016; Wilson 2018), and some bereaved mothers experience milk donation as part of their healing process following infant loss (Carroll et al 2014; Carroll and Lenne 2019; Oreg 2019). Transmasculine individuals – people who are assigned female at birth but who identify as male – may also become peer milk donors during lactation after giving birth, or may become recipients as a result of physical complications producing milk, such as in the case of chest surgery, or social discomfort with chestfeeding (MacDonald et al 2016; Giles 2017; Wilson 2018).

Peer breastmilk sharing in the contemporary Global North exists at the intersection of compliance and defiance of biomedical infant-feeding recommendations, and the medicalization and demedicalization of breastfeeding and breastmilk (Gribble 2014a; Palmquist 2015; Falls 2017; Shaw and Morgan 2017; Carter et al 2018). Medical organizations and public health campaigns promote exclusive breastfeeding for at least the first six months, citing biomedical research supporting the nutritional and immunological benefits of breastmilk compared with infant formula, and using slogans such as 'breast is best' (Wall 2001; Knaak 2006; Kukla 2006; Jansson 2009; Wolf 2010). Parents and other caregivers choose to donate or receive peer breastmilk because they believe that breastmilk is healthier for babies than its artificial substitutes, and they draw on biomedical and scientific discourses to substantiate their beliefs (Gribble 2013; Palmquist 2015; Carter et al 2018; Cassar-Uhl and Liberatos 2018; McCloskey and Karandikar 2019). Our research (Carter et al 2018) shows that milk-sharing participants tend to view mothers' own milk as slightly healthier than peer-shared milk, although they view both forms of human milk as significantly healthier than formula. They draw on biomedical and scientific discourses to substantiate their beliefs, criticizing the artificiality of infant formula and questioning the healthiness of its ingredients. Although they tend to report that mothers' own milk is specially formulated for their own babies' unique needs, and therefore is not a perfect fit for a recipient baby, their overall perceptions can be captured with the phrase they repeated throughout our study, 'breast is best, donor next'. Thus, although peer milk sharing violates FDA and AAP recommendations against feeding breastmilk acquired directly from individuals or over the internet, it simultaneously reflects hyper-adherence to recommendations by AAP and other public health agencies to feed babies breastmilk rather than formula. Further, participants modified the 'breast is best' slogan, popularized by breastfeeding advocacy groups and public health campaigns, to create a new version that promotes peer milk sharing. Aunchalee Palmquist (2015) argues that peer milk sharing occupies a liminal space between medicalization and demedicalization, and as such reliance on scientific and biomedical understandings of breastmilk to inform milk sharing practices reiterates the medicalization of breastmilk and breastfeeding, while the simultaneous circumventing of biomedical institutions reflects demedicalization.

Some critics of peer milk sharing argue that caregivers who are unable to provide their own breastmilk should acquire human milk from milk banks, although most peer milk recipients are ineligible, as banked milk is reserved for fragile infants, and commonly distributed to those in NICUs (Bar-Yam 2010; Swanson 2011; Gribble 2013). Regardless of eligibility, some peer milk-sharing participants critique the pasteurization process human milk undergoes in milk banks, reporting that some of the healthy bacteria and immunological benefits are eliminated through this processing (Gribble 2014a). Formal definitions of milk kinship such as those in Muslim cultures preclude the donor anonymity that is maintained at milk banks, making peer milk sharing more desirable for parents of certain cultural backgrounds

(Shaikh and Ahmed 2006; Cassidy and El Tom 2010; Ramli and Ibrahim 2010; Gribble 2013). Some peer milk donors select peer donation over donating to a milk bank because they prefer helping members of their own communities and want to know who is receiving their milk (Gribble 2013). This preference for sharing milk among peers rather than through formalized biomedical institutions reflects the demedicalization of breastmilk, as exchanges of human milk are coordinated outside of biomedical supervision (Palmquist 2015).

Yet, milk-sharers engage with medicalized views of breastmilk in their attempts to manage the perceived risks involved in peer milk sharing (Thorley 2012; Gribble 2014a; Palmquist 2015; Palmquist and Doehler 2016; Reyes-Foster et al 2017). Karleen Gribble's (2014a) research shows that recipients are aware of some of the reported potential risks involved in peer milk sharing, including drug or bacterial contamination and spread of infectious diseases. Recipients take actions to minimize risks by screening their donors for use of substances such as caffeine, alcohol or medications, requesting medical records, and establishing relationships based on mutual trust. Trust is a critical component of peer milk-sharing relationships, as it fosters confidence in the quality of milk among recipients and assures donors that their breastmilk is appreciated and used appropriately by recipients (Cassidy 2012a, 2012b; Gribble 2014a, 2914c, 2018; Palmquist 2015; Falls 2017; Shaw and Morgan 2017; Reyes-Foster and Carter 2018a, 2018b). Gribble's (2014a) study found that most donors identify no risks to themselves in giving milk, whereas some describe meeting a stranger as a potential danger or express concerns over liability if a problem were to occur with their milk. Most donors work to ensure the health and safety of the breastmilk they donate by washing and sterilizing equipment and storage containers, washing their hands, and promptly freezing their milk (Gribble 2014a), and donors and recipients in our study reported largely complying with the ABM's clinical recommendations for breastmilk handling and storage (Reyes-Foster et al 2017). Such adherence demonstrates that peer milk sharers do not reject medicalized views of breastmilk, but instead that breastmilk sharing reflects both the medicalization and demedicalization of breastmilk and breastfeeding, and the simultaneous rejection and hyper-adherence to biomedical infant feeding recommendations (Gribble 2014a; Palmquist 2015; Falls 2017; Shaw and Morgan 2017; Carter et al 2018).

Although the internet provides the capacity to connect people across the world, most peer milk sharing – even when facilitated online – takes place within local communities (Cassidy 2012a; Gribble 2013, 2014a; Reyes-Foster et al 2015, 2017; Palmquist and Doehler 2016;

Falls 2017; Reyes-Foster and Carter 2018c). Most caregivers meet in person to transfer milk from donor to recipient, and very few ever send milk through the mail (Reyes-Foster et al 2015, 2017; Palmquist and Doehler 2016). Most peer milk is transferred without monetary compensation, as there are strong taboos against the sale and purchase of human milk within peer milk-sharing communities, and monetary exchange for breastmilk is strictly prohibited by Human Milk 4 Human Babies and Eats on Feets (Cassidy 2012a, 2012b; Gribble 2014a, 2014b, 2014c; Palmquist and Doehler 2014, 2016; Palmquist 2015; Reyes-Foster et al 2015; Shaw 2015, 2019; Falls 2017; Shaw and Morgan 2017; Carter et al 2018; O'Sullivan et al 2018; Reyes-Foster and Carter 2018a, 2018b; Wilson 2018). These practices are also presumed to ensure the quality of peer-shared milk, as meeting in person is often part of the screening process for recipients and rejecting monetary compensation for breastmilk removes incentives to manipulate the volume of milk to increase profits.

Beyond infant feeding

Although the purpose of peer milk sharing may be to provide human milk to infants, the practice has significant individual and social outcomes beyond infant feeding. Peer milk sharing can foster a positive maternal identity for donors and recipients, providing new pathways for meeting breastfeeding goals and establishing support networks (Gribble 2014a, 2014b, 2018; Palmquist 2015; Shaw and Morgan 2017). Many who use peer breastmilk are mothers who are committed to breastfeeding but experience insufficient milk supply (Palmquist and Doehler 2014, 2016; Perrin et al 2014; Falls 2017). One study found that among mothers with low milk supply, those who supplemented with peer-shared milk were more likely to breastfeed longer and report greater satisfaction with their supplementation choices than those who did not supplement with peer-shared milk (Cassar-Uhl and Liberatos 2018). Nourishing one's baby with human milk creates a sense of relief and comfort and reduces self-reported postpartum depression and anxiety among mothers who experience breastfeeding difficulties (McCloskey and Karandikar 2019). Because breastfeeding is commonly associated with 'good mothering' in the Global North, especially according to white middle- and upper-class heterosexual archetypes (Marshall et al 2007; Knaak 2010; Ryan et al 2010; Stearns 2010; Carter 2017; Lee 2018a), using peer breastmilk helps mothers affirm their identities as moral mothers – individuals who adhere to dominant idealized notions of motherhood – especially when they prove themselves to be hardworking neoliberal subjects by working hard to feed their babies breastmilk despite adverse circumstances (Shaw and Morgan 2017; Reyes-Foster and Carter 2018a, 2018b).

Although non-reciprocated giving, where one makes a sacrifice for the good of another without expecting anything in return, is commonly viewed as an altruistic act, social scientists have long challenged this perspective (Mauss 1950 [1925]; Comte 1974 [1855]; Strathern 1990). In contrast to the view of breastfeeding as self-sacrifice, Fiona Giles conceptualizes breastfeeding as an act of 'self-care' that 'provides an analogy for the gift of connection which benefits both parties' (2010: 242). Similarly, donating breastmilk, whether to a milk bank or directly to peers, provides donors with a sense of personal satisfaction and pride, fostering a 'good mothering' identity (Shaw 2010, 2019; Carroll 2015; Shaw and Morgan 2017; Gribble 2018; Reyes-Foster and Carter 2018b). Many donors benefit by feeling good about their giving, describing themselves as feeling 'happy to be able to help' (Gribble 2014b), and donating milk is particularly beneficial for supporting a maternal identity following infant loss (Carroll and Lenne 2019; Oreg 2019).

Peer milk sharing also facilitates interpersonal relationships. Many donors and recipients report that establishing relationships is an important part of milk sharing, even when initial contact is established over the internet (Gribble 2018). Although not essential, many donor–recipient pairs arrange playdates or attend birthday parties, and some develop close friendships. Recipients often view these relationships as significant for establishing trust, whereas for donors, relationships provide incentive to continue expressing milk for a recipient baby (Falls 2017; Gribble 2018). Beyond the milk kinship formally recognized by Islamic law (Cassidy and El Tom 2010; Ramli and Ibrahim 2010), some participants consider milk sharing to form the basis of familial relationships, identifying children who have consumed the same mother's milk as 'milk siblings' or establishing close emotional ties between the donor and recipient child (Thorley 2014; Gribble 2018; Wilson 2018). Kristin Wilson calls these 'affective relations' because they are based on emotional ties rather than the blood, marriage, or adoption that traditionally defines family ties, yet the relationships differ from friendship. As Wilson states, 'They become bonded not by blood but by milk' (2018: 188). Expanding more broadly, Tanya Cassidy and Abdullahi El Tom (2010) describe the sense of 'imagined community' experienced when receiving milk from a milk bank, even though these donors are anonymous. This sense of connectedness and feelings of gratitude toward others who share milk, whether they are known or unknown, in one's own community or across the world, is also characteristic of peer milk sharing (Falls 2017; Shaw and Morgan 2017; Shaw 2019).

Peer milk sharing has broader societal and global implications. Consuming human milk is shown to have numerous short- and long-term benefits, and therefore is often included in national objectives for improving population health. Because supplementing with donor milk is shown to increase breastfeeding longevity among mothers with low milk supply, Diana Cassar-Uhl and Penny Liberatos (2018) argue that peer milk sharing can help nations meet their goals, including the US Healthy People 2030 Objectives. Peer milk sharing can also be viewed as a 'global movement' (Cassidy 2012a), holding the potential to substantially increase the global supply of human milk, thereby improving infant health worldwide (Akre et al 2011).

Methods

Birth and breastfeeding in Central Florida

Our research took place in Central Florida, a region spanning the urban centre of Orlando and surrounding suburbs, smaller towns and rural areas outside the city, and beach towns that line the Atlantic Ocean. Breastfeeding in this region is fairly typical of the US, with breastfeeding initiation and duration rates for the state of Florida just slightly below the national average (CDC 2018) (see Table 1.1). Although Florida tends to lean socially and politically conservative on the whole, the greater Orlando Metropolitan Area is socially and politically mixed, comprising around two million residents who are diverse in terms of racial, ethnic and socioeconomic status. James Wright and Amy Donley highlight that Orlando is largely typical of other industrial areas, characterizing it as 'a metaphor for the twenty-first century post-industrial city' (2011: 6), with sprawling city suburbs.

Table 1.1: Breastfeeding initiation and duration rates in the US and Florida

	Initiation	**Breastfeeding at six months**	**Exclusive breastfeeding at six months**	**Breastfeeding at 12 months**
US	83.2%	57.6%	24.9%	35.9%
Florida	82.6%	54.0%	21.3%	33.5%

Source: CDC 2018

Central Florida offers a wide range of maternity care and breastfeeding support services. In Orange and Seminole Counties, where much of our research took place, there are five hospitals that offer maternity services, three free-standing birth centres and several home-birth midwives. Some midwives accept regular health insurance, including Medicaid, making out-of-hospital birth widely accessible throughout the region. Orlando and surrounding areas also offer five public health centres that provide prenatal care and ten Women, Infants and Children (WIC) offices, many of which provide lactation services. There are a variety of other breastfeeding services available, with at least five active La Leche League chapters with monthly support groups, five additional weekly or bi-weekly breastfeeding support groups, and at least ten annual events centered on breastfeeding and infant care. Many of the breastfeeding support groups operate private groups on Facebook, where parents can share breastfeeding information and support. Several local groups and organizations promote parenting practices other than breastfeeding including baby wearing, cloth diapering and natural parenting more generally. These groups may exist online, meet face to face, or both, and often attract overlapping membership. As our research shows, many milk-sharing relationships are established through participation in these groups that are created for purposes other than to facilitate milk sharing. There are also state-wide Facebook pages for Eats on Feets and Human Milk 4 Human Babies, where participants can post a request to receive or donate milk to someone in their local region.

Central Florida houses a local, non-profit, milk-sharing organization, Get Pumped. Get Pumped collects breastmilk from screened donors and distributes it to parents who are unable to otherwise provide exclusive breastmilk to their babies. Get Pumped uses donor screening guidelines similar to those used by HMBANA-affiliated milk banks to determine eligibility of breastmilk donors, including a health and diet questionnaire, blood test for communicable diseases, and precise instructions on expressing and handling breastmilk. However, unlike HMBANA-affiliated milk banks, the organization does not test or process the milk. Recipients also complete a screening process that asks information about the circumstances leading to the request and other potential sources of human milk. Approved recipients pick up unprocessed, frozen milk from various locations (such as local businesses and health provider offices) that serve as collection/distribution sites and receive information on how to pasteurize the milk themselves. The organization requests a donation of US$1 per ounce to cover their operating costs and to pay for donor blood-screening tests. Several reproductive healthcare providers in the region provide drop-off and pick-up locations for Get Pumped, and some operate their own informal breastmilk transfers between their patients.

When we officially began our research in 2013, there were no HMBANA-affiliated milk banks in the region. However, in 2015, Mothers' Milk Bank of Florida opened its doors. Like other HMBANA-affiliated milk banks, Mothers' Milk Bank of Florida distributes processed breastmilk primarily to NICUs. Given the constraints on access to banked milk described earlier, the opening of the milk bank did not appear to affect peer milk sharing in the region. Similar to previous research showing that milk donors typically either donate to milk banks or to peers, but not both (Gribble 2013; Perrin et al 2016), none of our participants donated to Mothers' Milk Bank of Florida. Nevertheless, we and some of our participants demonstrated support for the milk bank by participating in annual fundraisers and occasional volunteer work. Likewise, the milk bank did not appear to falter as a result of peer milk sharing in the region, as the staff described receiving generous donations of milk from local donors, and the bank has been filled with donated milk whenever we or our students have volunteered to help process it.

Data collection and analysis

This research is based on an in-depth ethnographic investigation of peer milk-sharing communities in Central Florida. Our interest in uncovering the practical, relational and symbolic aspects of peer milk sharing, as well as revealing the influential impact of the milk itself, fuelled our data collection techniques. We utilized aspects of actor–network theory, which is a 'material-semiotic' approach that considers the impact of materiality as well as language and meanings in the assembling of social phenomena (Latour 2005; Law 2009), to guide our research design. To this end, we employed ethnographic techniques that attended to the social components of peer milk sharing and the physical materiality of the milk itself (Carter and Reyes-Foster 2020).

Our data are derived from four years of ethnographic engagement, an online survey, and 33 semi-structured qualitative interviews. We have engaged in participant observation of milk-sharing communities in Central Florida since autumn 2013. Participation observation is a qualitative methodology commonly used in cultural anthropology and sociology that requires researchers to become immersed in the daily life of the communities they study, a prolonged period of rapprochement, and engagement that frequently results in the development of long-term relationships (Emerson and Fretz 2001). Both study authors were mothers of nursing children during part of the time this research was conducted. This common interest facilitated rapport and acceptance into the communities. During the course of our own lactation, we participated in various breastfeeding support groups that met weekly and took part in other meet-ups related to natural birth, natural parenting, cloth diapering and baby wearing. Throughout the study period, we attended and facilitated various local activities, including Big Latch On events, Great Cloth Diaper Changes, parenting and baby expos, and social events hosted by local midwives, the Central Florida chapter of the International Cesarean Awareness Network (ICAN), Get Pumped, and The Breastfeeding Project. We formed partnerships with local birth, parenting, breastfeeding and milk-sharing organizations and frequented breastfeeding support groups and events where milk-sharing relationships often develop. We also established a positive relationship with Mothers' Milk Bank of Florida by participating in its annual fundraising event, volunteering at the milk bank, and arranging for our students to volunteer through our student organization at the University of Central Florida, Reproductive Justice Knights.

Our observational data collection techniques focused on interactions among milk-sharing participants, the social networks and relationships they established, and the ways they handled and interacted with the milk. We focused on the practices involved in peer milk sharing and the meanings associated with the milk and its alternatives (mothers' own milk or infant formula). Following our actor–network approach (Carter and Reyes-Foster 2020), we also 'followed the milk' as it was produced and expressed by a donor, through its handling and transfer to a peer recipient, and ultimately to the recipient parent feeding it to their baby. Although our participant observation was carried out in person, many interactions took place in online communities of which we were members, including local 'mommy groups' on Facebook. Members of the community knew we were researchers and mothers of nursing children from a local university studying human milk sharing, and we were able to use these online networks to recruit participants for our survey and interviews. We encountered a community eager to have its voice heard. Participants readily volunteered to share their stories with us and connect us with others in their networks. This became particularly noticeable when we developed our survey, as we received over 200 responses in the first month alone. Later, when our early publications received media attention, the articles and news clips were highly circulated among our participant communities.

Our survey consisted of a total of 102 closed- and open-ended questions, containing quantifiable multiple-choice and Likert-scale questions as well as qualitative questions. Question sets were asked to participants depending on the nature of their involvement in peer milk sharing (for example, as donors, recipients or both, or in cross-nursing arrangements, and so on). We developed and administered our survey using the survey program Qualtrics. We recruited participants through distribution of our survey link through Facebook in 18 private Central Florida breastfeeding, mothering and milk-sharing groups, the Florida pages of Eat on Feets and Human Milk 4 Human Babies, our own personal pages, and the pages of 20 professional contacts (lactation counsellors, breastfeeding advocates, midwives and alternative medicine practitioners) who assisted with recruitment. Once the survey link was initially distributed, it was reshared by other page members to their personal networks, making it difficult to trace the exact number of times the link was shared. We also recruited participants by distributing study flyers at local breastfeeding support meetings, family events and baby expos with support from a local breastfeeding advocacy and education organization, The Breastfeeding Project. A total of 350 printed flyers were distributed with the survey website address. Approximately one third of our survey sample resided in areas of the US outside the target region. These participants are included in our analysis because independent analyses found no significant differences between the two groups.

When a potential participant gained entry into the online survey, they were presented with a prompt as follows: 'Milk sharing is the exchange of human milk including cross-feeding (also known as wet nursing) and exchanging expressed milk (including direct exchange, donation to a milk bank or organization like Get Pumped).[4] A milk-sharing participant is one who has given, received or facilitated milk sharing. Have you ever participated in milk sharing?' If the respondent answered 'yes', they could take the survey. All participants were asked questions about their milk-sharing practices, perceptions of milk sharing, and demographic characteristics. The survey was distributed from April 2014 to September 2014 and took approximately 30 minutes to complete.

In addition to the online survey, we conducted 30 in-depth, semi-structured interviews with caretakers in Central Florida who were engaged in milk sharing as donors or recipients at the time of the interviews. Participants were recruited through online social networking and snowball sampling. Interviews were conducted between August and October 2015. All interviews were conducted by Shannon or Beatriz (we also sometimes conducted interviews together) and took place in person at a location of the participants' choosing, most often their home or a local coffee shop. Interviews were semi-structured, where we followed a general interview schedule, but allowed the interviews to flow in a conversational manner and provided participants the ability to discuss issues they found important outside of the questions on our schedule. The schedules contained questions about milk-sharing practices, milk-sharing relationships, milk handling, and personal convictions about breastmilk compared with formula use, use of donor milk and its safety, and the commodification of breastmilk. We also asked participants about the physical objects and spaces they used in their milk-sharing practices, and when interviews took place in participants' homes, they showed us where their milk-sharing practices occurred and the objects that mediated it. Interviews lasted, on average, 40 minutes to one hour.

We also conducted three in-depth, semi-structured interviews with healthcare providers and organizational leaders in Central Florida involved in peer milk sharing. We used purposive sampling techniques to identify participants who were involved in milk sharing in different ways. The sample of healthcare providers included lactation consultants and midwives who worked with individuals engaged in milk sharing and facilitated it in some way, and had various levels of involvement with the local organization Get Pumped. All interviews were audio recorded and transcribed verbatim, and all interview participants chose their own pseudonyms for anonymity in publications.[5]

Qualitative interview data and observational field notes were analyzed inductively to identify common and uncommon themes in the practice of peer milk sharing. We began with an open coding process (Charmaz and Belgrave 2012) where each author independently reviewed several transcripts and sets of field notes and generated a list of themes. Based on existing research on milk sharing, ongoing controversies surrounding the safety of the practice, and our material-semiotic approach, we approached our analysis with particular interest in topics concerning participants' perceptions and practices related to the health and safety of milk sharing, the meanings and relationships that formed through milk sharing, and the role of the milk itself. As themes developed, we engaged in focused coding (Charmaz and Belgrave 2012) to organize data into themes and subthemes to identify patterns and nuances in the data. Quantitative survey data were analyzed in Qualtrics and SPSS to identify broad patterns in milk-sharing practices, such as demographic characteristics, practices of cross-nursing or transferring frozen milk, and health and safety perceptions. Qualitative survey data were analyzed in Microsoft Excel to facilitate the organization of open-ended data into themes. The survey data provided a broad overview of milk sharing based on a larger sample size, whereas the interview and observational data provided richness and depth into individuals' personal experiences of the practice.

The sample

The sample culled from the online survey consisted of 392 individuals who participated in peer breastmilk sharing.[6] Although all survey respondents had participated in milk sharing at some point in time, not all were still engaged in the practice. In contrast, all individuals who participated in our ethnographic interviews resided in Central Florida and were actively engaged in milk sharing at the time the interview took place. Both groups were predominantly white, cisgender, heterosexual, married, and in middle- and upper-middle income brackets, and had some college education. In other words, the sample is characterized by a high degree of racial and socioeconomic privilege with access to cultural and social capital.

Among survey participants, 61.2% were breastmilk donors, 24.2% were breastmilk recipients, and 17.6% had both donated and received peer breastmilk. Among donors, 80.4% reported only donating expressed milk and 19.2% reported both donating expressed milk and co-feeding. Among recipients, 86.7% reported only receiving expressed milk and 13.3% reported having their child cross-fed and receiving expressed milk. Only one donor (0.04%) and no recipients reported only participating in co-feeding (Reyes-Foster et al 2015). See Appendix A for more information on survey participants' demographic characteristics.

The interview sample consisted of 30 individuals who participated in peer milk sharing and three maternity care providers who were involved with milk-sharing participants or facilitated milk sharing in some way. The milk-sharing participants interviewed all identified as cisgender, heterosexual women who were mothers, and who participated in milk sharing as part of their role as parents. All resided in Central Florida at the time of interview. They were predominantly white, married or cohabiting, with some college education, and one or two children. Most identified as Christian, and although religion emerges as an impetus for milk sharing for a few participants, it was not a driving force for most, and seven identified as having no religious affiliation or being agnostic. Among interviewees, 20 engaged in milk sharing only as donors, seven participated as recipients, and three were both donors and recipients, typically at different points in their childbearing careers. See Appendix B for more information on interview participants' demographic characteristics. To protect anonymity, we did not collect specific demographic information from healthcare providers.

Making sense of milk sharing

Sharing Milk comprises six chapters outlining our theoretical approach and analysis of peer milk sharing in the US as it occurs throughout the Central Florida communities studied. Having provided the contextual background of our research in Chapter 1, in Chapter 2 we present the theoretical underpinnings of our book. We build on theories of situated learning, biological citizenship and biovalue to arrive at the concept of bio-communities of practice as a framework for understanding peer breastmilk sharing. We argue that peer milk-sharing communities can be conceptualized as bio-communities of practice where bio-intimacy is created through the exchange of biological material and the establishing of (bio-)intimacy and affective bonds between donors and recipients.

In Chapter 3, we examine the process of becoming part of milk sharing bio-communities of practice, exploring the journeys of people who have encountered milk sharing as donors and recipients. We explore the primary circumstances through which people come to give milk or seek it out for their babies, and how milk sharing participants become socialized into their bio-communities of practice. Subsequently, Chapter 4 provides a detailed analysis of milk-sharing practices, 'following the milk' as it makes its way from the bodies of donors through the bodies of recipient infants. We consider the body work and embodied labour of making and expressing milk, its management, handling and storage, and the ways in which donors and recipients find each other. Finally, we consider the effects of shared milk on the bodies of the babies who consume it.

In Chapter 5, we take a step back to consider the functioning of breastmilk sharing in society. We explore the foundational context from which milk sharing emerges, the online and offline social networks that enable its existence, and the role of certain key actors in facilitating milk-sharing relationships. Through this process, bio-intimacy and bio-connectedness develop between people who participate in milk sharing, establishing and maintaining bio-communities of practice. Finally, in Chapter 6, we consider the greater implications of our project, particularly in policy and practice and in its potential for presenting an alternative way of understanding social connectedness.

2

Theorizing Milk Sharing

I (Beatriz) met Anna in her modest apartment in Casselberry, a middle-income community in Central Florida. She opened the door holding six-month-old Grace, a beautiful baby girl with twinkling blue eyes. Anna was young, only 21, younger than most of the women who had participated in our study. When her baby girl was born, Anna was a single mother, working two minimum-wage jobs to support herself and her baby. Her story was harrowing: she explained that although she had been planning a vaginal birth, she experienced complications that led to a caesarean section (C-section). She qualified for Medicaid and thus had health insurance; however, like most women in the US, she did not have access to paid maternity leave, and her wages were very low. So, even though she was still physically recovering from major surgery, and even though her infant daughter was still very young, Anna had no choice but to return to work only 15 days after giving birth.

Anna firmly believes that human milk is the best possible nutrition for her baby. When Grace was born, nearly everything that could go wrong did go wrong: Grace was taken from Anna during the C-section and not returned to her for 90 minutes, despite Anna being promised that she would be able to have skin-to-skin contact with Grace in the operating room. Then Grace developed jaundice and had to be hospitalized. For four days, Anna slept in the hospital lobby, getting up every two hours to go to the NICU to nurse her baby.

Things got harder once Anna was able to bring Grace home. She knew federal law guaranteed her the right to express her milk, and that her employer was required to give her a space to do so. But she knew that because she held an unskilled job and worked for low wages her position was vulnerable. Her supervisor agreed to give her breaks so she could pump, but there was no space for her to do it at the gas station where she worked, so she had to do it in her car. Whenever she went out to her car to pump, she endured ridicule, harassment and snide remarks from coworkers who resented the breaks she was receiving. If things got busy, she couldn't always take the time to go out to her car to pump. She developed a thyroid condition that further compromised her ability to produce enough milk for Grace. Her breastmilk supply began to dwindle, and baby Grace wasn't gaining weight. Overwhelmed and devastated, Anna decided to seek out donor milk.

Soon, she found herself spending hours on end scouring the Facebook pages of Human Milk 4 Human Babies, Eats on Feets and a few local natural parenting groups. As soon as she saw an offer of milk, she would immediately pursue it. She posted ads requesting milk, sharing pictures of baby Grace to get the attention of potential donors.[1] The offers started coming in, and Anna never turned one down. When she wasn't working, she spent hours on the road, driving long distances, collecting milk and bringing it home. She figured out the best way to transport it and the most efficient ways to keep it frozen, and she emptied out her freezer to make room for breastmilk. She showed me her 'stash', beaming, a freezer full of frozen bags of milk. "[When] my freezer's full, I'm happy, I feel like it's Christmas!," she said. She picked one bag up and held it. I took her picture. She explained that, along her journey, she developed relationships with several regular donors, and also took many donations from people she only ever met once. All in all, she estimated, baby Grace had received milk from over 30 donors.

Describing her process, Anna talked about driving long distances, sometimes as far as the Florida coast, to pick up milk. Pulling a large black bag that resembled a pizza delivery bag out of her closet, Anna opened it to reveal the insulated interior. "This is my lifesaver bag," she explained, "I fill it with five, six hundred ounces of milk and bring it home. It keeps it frozen until I get here."

Anna used every drop of milk she could. She explained:

> 'I've noticed a lot of my bags leak and I do not want to waste any milk. So, I usually put it in a big cake pan. I usually rinse the bags off just to make sure there's no dirt on it etcetera and then I put it in the baking pan and then I let it defrost a little to where I can pour it in another container. I put them outside on the counter and then when they defrost, they're still a little freezing cold, so it would be higher than a refrigerator temperature is what I would assume. I put them in another container if they're leaking and if they're not I rinse off the bags and put them in the fridge. And I have Ziploc bags at the bottom of my fridge so they're

> not in the door, so if they do leak – I don't know if this is necessarily sanitary but in my opinion it's all good – if the bags did leak in the baking pan I pour what's in the baking pan in another cup. So, I've rinsed off the bags, and I mean, it's not like the bags were thrown in dirt. She's alright, builds her immune system. If there's a dirt speck in there she'll be okay. But I honestly believe in no milk being wasted at all. Like, people say, "Oh is she done with this bottle? I'll just throw it in the sink," and I say, "No, no, no! That bottle's good. She'll be fine."'

Anna recognized that some might object to the way she tried to save milk from waste by collecting leaked milk in a cake pan or storing her bags inside a larger plastic bag to collect leaked milk. As she explains, going through these extraordinary measures reduces potential waste and, in the end, having her daughter receive as much human milk as possible outweighed any risk of potential harm in her milk handling methods.[2]

Anna's story highlights the ways milk sharing encompasses an array of embodied and social practices. To begin with, Anna undergoes a traumatic bodily experience of childbirth followed by structural obstacles to her breastfeeding relationship. Then, she must spend significant energy searching for donors, ultimately developing relationships – some temporary, some long-lasting – that enable her to successfully feed her daughter human milk. Finally, the milk itself has an important material presence in her story as she describes the ways she transports, stores and handles it, alongside the deep emotional connection she experiences with it. Through Anna, we can see human milk sharing as community, (embodied) practice and material. These various aspects of milk sharing form the theoretical groundwork for our book. We build on Étienne Wenger's communities of practice model to propose the notion of bio-communities of practice, which, although formed through practice, are characterized by bio-intimacy (Shaw and Morgan 2017; Shaw 2019). Bio-intimacy is also interconnected with the materiality of human milk, particularly the ways in which it is an emotionally laden substance. We further develop this framework to account for the 'emotional materiality' of milk. In so doing, we build on existing scholarship, aiming to understand the communities and relationships that constitute and are constituted by peer breastmilk sharing (Cassidy 2012a, 2012b; Thorley 2012; Gribble 2014b, 2018; Perrin et al 2014; Palmquist 2015; Falls 2017; Shaw and Morgan 2017; Wilson 2018; Shaw 2019).

Communities of practice

Communities of practice is a conceptual model developed by Wenger and colleagues (Lave 1991; Lave and Wenger 1991; Wenger 1998, 2010; Wenger and Snyder 2000), which can be defined as groups of people brought together by a common goal or practice. Communities of practice are formal or informal groups whose members come together and engage in collective learning that leads to practices which reflect their social relations and are pursuant of a specific goal. A community of practice can be a family, a group of individuals who work together at a particular job, graduate students within a programme who work in proximity to each other, or participants of a breastfeeding support group. The individuals who make up the community of practice do not come together intentionally to form a community, but rather to achieve a specific goal: to earn a living, acquire a college degree, or feed their babies breastmilk. Although originally developed to understand how individuals and groups come together through face-to-face interactions to form and sustain communities of practice, the concept has more recently been applied to online interactions (Wasko and Faraj 2000; Johnson 2001). Continual, ongoing interaction is necessary to keep individuals engaged in online communities of practice, and through engagement they feel a sense of personal attachment and commitment to the group.

The milk-sharing groups we observed fit well within the communities of practice model. Most participated in milk sharing with the goal of feeding breastmilk to their own or to others' babies and young children. They did not come together purposefully to form a community, and they varied on whether they thought milk sharers made up a community or not. Moreover, the communities of practice model conceptualizes these communities as loosely structured and flexible in membership. This flexibility is visible in milk sharing, due to the fact that the lactation period is time-limited. As Mary Bucholtz (1996) observed in her study of a community of nerd girls in southern California, the communities of practice model allows participants to set boundaries of the community internally, rather than having boundaries imposed externally by researchers.

Communities of practice have been purposefully implemented as an intentional strategy to facilitate peer-to-peer learning in business, education and healthcare settings, and have been identified as emerging organically in many organizational and community situations. In healthcare, communities of practice have been deliberately established for providers to facilitate education, promote collaboration across disciplines or professional expertise, and improve patient care (Ranmuthugala et al 2011). Communities of practice are also created by practitioners for their patients to share experiential knowledge about specific health issues, such as chronic illness and pain management (Winkelman and Choo 2003; Meins et al 2015). In reproductive healthcare, organizational establishment of communities of practice among maternity care patients has been shown in clinical trials to have positive outcomes, such as increasing rates of vaginal birth after cesarean (VBAC) (Clarke et al 2015). Patient and provider communities of practice are often established virtually in order to promote efficiency of communication, reach underserved populations, and connect individuals who are immobile or geographically distant (Struminger et al 2017). Thus, the communities of practice model can be employed as a strategic method for expanding learning among professionals to encourage collaboration across disciplines or professional expertise. It is also a phenomenon that emerges organically among healthcare consumers to share information about healthcare practices, resources and service providers. It is within the latter that we situate peer milk-sharing groups as communities of practice.

Situated learning

The communities of practice model was originally developed as a way of understanding situated learning. From this perspective, learning is a social process that takes place in the context of everyday life (Wenger 1999). As individuals interact with others in social contexts, they gain knowledge about how things are done in the social setting and gain competence in these activities. They use their knowledge to actively engage in the world, and in so doing, they produce meanings. Thus, practice, identity, meaning and community are interconnected components of social learning. The communities of practice model is based on, but not limited to, a Bourdieuan understanding of practice. Where for Bourdieu (1990), learning is an individuated process whereby the social becomes inscribed on to the body of the person through practices that become embodied knowledge or habitus, communities of practice builds on this notion to consider how learning takes place within groups.

Within the communities of practice model, practice consists of both process and meaning. Wenger explains practice as 'a process by which we can experience the world and our engagement with it as meaningful' (1999: 52). Consistent with contemporary sociological and anthropological approaches, the meanings of practices are not static, but instead are negotiated with others who participate in the community of practice. Individuals within the group engage in certain practices because of what those practices mean to them, and they learn, employ and modify the meanings of practices through their participation. The negotiation of meanings within practices involves the duality of participation and reification, whereby individuals take part in processes with others, and through their participation they develop words, concepts, stories and documents that reify – or make tangible – the processes they engage in.

Viewing milk sharing within the communities of practice model led us to consider the role of labour. As we discussed earlier, the communities of practice model is based on a Bourdieuan notion of practice. Although he is building on the work of Karl Marx, Bourdieu moves away from labour to focus on practice. Within his approach, one could argue that all labour is practice; however, not all practice is labour. As feminist scholars, we argue that milk-sharing practices, like breastfeeding (Law 2000; Bartlett 2002; Stearns 2009, 2010, 2013; Hausman 2014), are always labour. Whereas Marx (1967 [1867]) distinguished productive labour – work that takes place in the paid labour sphere – from reproductive labour – predominantly unpaid work that takes place within the home to reproduce the species and maintain the human population – feminist scholars such as Ann Oakley (1974 [2019], 1976, 2018), Mariarosa Dalla Costa and Selma James (1972) and Heidi Hartmann (1976) have critiqued this distinction. It is not only based on heteropatriarchal assumptions of public/private separation and a (cis)gendered division of labour, but it contributes to the devaluation of the significant contributions, paid and unpaid, that women and other non-male individuals make to society, and the embodied and intellectual work required for these contributions.

Our conceptualization of milk-sharing practices as labour is consistent with previous social science scholarship that views the processes of breastfeeding one's own child, and expressing and donating milk, as work (Law 2000; Bartlett 2002; Avishai 2007; Stearns 2009, 2010; Carroll 2014, 2015; Hausman 2014). This scholarship highlights the bodily effort involved in breastfeeding, which stands in contrast to dominant portrayals of breastfeeding as a 'natural' process that occurs without any effort or training (Locke 2009; Carter 2017). Cindy A. Stearns (1999, 2009) argues that opposition to public breastfeeding delegates this labour-intensive aspect of motherhood to the home, keeping such labour hidden from public view. This mandate to keep breastfeeding labour hidden is often even more pronounced in African American families and communities (Blum 1999; Owens et al 2018). Likewise, norms defining pumping milk as a private act (Stearns 2010) and breastmilk sharing as subversive practice make the labour involved in donating and receiving peer milk private, and therefore invisible. Thus, our use of the conceptualization of the practices that make up peer milk sharing as labour contribute analysis to the visibility of this work.

The notion of individual social identities is also central to the concept of communities of practice (Wenger 1999). Individuals participate in communities of practice as social beings, taking part in the practices, and learning and modifying the meanings associated with them. However, they participate as individuals, with their own unique sets of previous experiences, skills, competencies and meanings, which are often derived from previous social experience (Blumer 1969). Becoming a member of the community of practice entails learning the practices and meanings of the group, which, in turn, alters the individual. Wenger explains, 'Learning is not just acquiring skills and information; it is becoming a certain person – a knower in a context where what it means to know is negotiated with respect to the regime of competence of a community' (2010: 181). Nevertheless, the community does not determine how individuals interpret, negotiate and modify the meanings and practices they learn from the community; instead, individuals maintain their dynamism as they establish their place within the community of practice. At the same time, learning within communities contributes to the refining of social practices and generation of new members.

Central characteristics

Communities of practice possess three central characteristics: 'mutual engagement', 'joint enterprise' and 'shared repertoire' (Wenger 1999). Mutual engagement is people engaged in practices that need not be identical but that are often complementary. Put simply, the practices exist because they are carried out by people. The community forms, not as a matter of similar identities or shared interests, but as a result of common practices, or mutual engagement. Mutual engagement leads to the establishment of relationships that emerge through participation in common or complementary practices. Milk-sharing communities develop because participants engage in the practices required for milk sharing to take place. Their mutual engagement – as donors, recipients and/or facilitators – renders the practice of peer milk sharing into existence.

Joint enterprise is the common or shared goal that participants in the community of practice come together to achieve (Wenger 1999). Joint enterprise is characterized by mutual accountability, where norms are established and negotiated. In this context, norms emerge through practices and are therefore able to be negotiated; they constrain practices, yet they do not determine them. Parents involved in milk sharing engage in the joint enterprise of making human milk available to babies who need it by either donating excess or receiving milk to feed their own child. All participants are mutually accountable for engaging in safe milk-sharing practices, yet they do not share identical interpretations of what this means. Rather, it is through mutual engagement and joint enterprise that rules and norms for what constitutes safe milk sharing are developed, negotiated, contested and reproduced.

Through mutual engagement and joint enterprise, communities of practice develop a shared repertoire, which includes 'routines, words, tools, ways of doing things, stories, gestures, symbols, genres, actions, or concepts that the community has produced or adopted in the course of its existence, and which have become part of its practice' (Wenger 1999: 83). Milk-sharing communities have a shared repertoire visible in the way participants talk about human milk and milk sharing, and follow spoken and unspoken rules about its practice. Participants consistently express the strong belief that human milk is the best possible food for human infants, reciting the well-known phrase 'breast is best', and their own modified version, 'breast is best, donor next'.[3] The shared repertoire reiterates the core values and shared meanings that drive the joint enterprise and are regularly communicated in online and offline forums.

The communities of practice model facilitates consideration of both central and peripheral participants (Lave and Wenger 1991). In milk sharing, this allows us to examine similarities and differences between a person who donates milk once by chance and another who makes a conscious effort to pump extra milk every day for the sole purpose of donating. In milk-sharing communities of practice, parents and other caregivers are finding each other and coming together, united by the goal of feeding human milk to human babies. In so doing, some form long-lasting relationships that outlive milk sharing as their children grow and wean. Others establish short-term relationships, sometimes only communicating or meeting once or twice.

Biological citizenship and bio-intimacy

Whereas a traditional breastfeeding support group where milk sharing does not occur can be read through the framework of communities of practice, milk sharing involves an added dimension – the sharing of biological material. Because US culture values notions of individual, bounded selfhood, the sharing of one's bodily products violates underlying cultural taboos (Shaw 2004a, 2015). The social processes involved in milk sharing require the development of trust and intimacy because breastfeeding itself is understood as a deeply intimate social practice (Shaw 2007, 2019; Cassidy 2012a, 2012b; Palmquist 2015; Tomori et al 2016; Falls 2017; Shaw and Morgan 2017; Gribble 2018; Reyes-Foster and Carter 2018a, 2018b; Wilson 2018). The intimacy of breastfeeding and the non-normative nature of human milk sharing necessitates the expansion of the communities of practice model.

Biological citizenship

Nikolas Rose and Carlos Novas (2005) coined the term 'biological citizenship' to describe the ways people come together around a biological experience. Building on Foucault's (1978) notion of 'biopower' and Rabinow's (1996) 'biosociality', Rose and Novas argue that lay engagement with biomedical and scientific knowledge is giving rise to new subjectivities and identity formations, giving people diagnosed with certain genetic conditions or illnesses such as AIDS a new sense of self as biological subjects. In turn, these newfound subjectivities bring people together to learn about their illness, share information, and at times engage in activism, building on notions of rights and citizenship to demand certain action from the state, such as making healthcare available or supporting biomedical research. Building on Rabinow's (1996) notion of biosociality, defined as the sociality created by a joint biological experience, biological citizens demand the state fulfill its mandate to promote the health and wellbeing of the population. Biological citizenship is an empowering concept, operating in a political economy of hope (Novas 2006). 'Contemporary biological citizenship, that is to say, is a hopeful domain of activity, one that depends upon and intensifies the hope that the science of the present will bring about cures or treatments in the near future' (Rose and Novas 2005: 441). Biological citizens thus trust in the potential of science and technology to better their lives.

A key characteristic of biological citizenship is that it is both individuating and collectivizing (Rose and Novas 2005). In this new regime of power, individuals are made responsible for managing their own health and wellbeing, and even their genome. By the same token, people are brought together by a shared biological subjectivity. In engaging in the management of their own biological selves through practices such as research, participation in support groups, and the deployment of technologies of knowledge such as the internet, the collectivizing effect of biological citizenship manifests. Through the internet and other forms of support networks, people come together to disseminate professional and experiential knowledge, forming the basis of political action. As conceptualized by Rose and Novas (2005), biological citizenship requires active political engagement. In many ways, biological citizenship is reminiscent of communities of practice.

To Rose and Novas (2005), biological citizenship comprises a contemporary regime of biopower. Biopower, originally developed in the work of Foucault (1978), refers to the way the state manages its population. Contemporary biopower operates through individuated governmentality, demanding citizens take personal responsibility for managing their health. Breastfeeding promotion by the state falls within the prerogative of this regime (Lee 2018a). Thus, the state promotes breastfeeding as the best infant nutrition and holds mothers responsible for national and global health objectives (Kukla 2006; Jansson 2009; Rippeyoung 2009; Waggoner 2011; Taylor and Wallace 2012). At the same time that national and global organizations have taken up the mantle of breastfeeding, some of these same entities undermine women's ability to meet their objectives by denying national, paid, parental leave and universal healthcare and by allowing the aggressive marketing of infant milk substitutes (Foss 2017). Moreover, the individuating operation of biopower feeds Euroamerican notions of the self as a bounded individual, limiting the definition of breastfeeding to that of a single mother feeding only her own infant. This limited definition of breastfeeding excludes other creative forms of breastfeeding, what Wilson (2018) calls exceptional breastfeeding practices. This includes cross-nursing and milk sharing, among others. Because caretakers have assumed the responsibility thrust on them by the state to breastfeed, they experience their inability or difficulty in breastfeeding as an individual failure of the body rather than the result of structurally imposed obstacles (Kelleher 2006; Stearns 2009; Ryan et al 2010).

According to Rose and Novas (2005), a primary characteristic of biological citizenship is that it operates within a 'political economy of hope'. Because of this and its inherent activist stance, one might argue that biological citizenship is an empowering framework.[4] This framework might be useful for thinking through social phenomena such as 'lactivism' (Faircloth 2013; Falls 2017; Wilson 2018), a movement that brings together parents, medical and lactation professionals, and breastfeeding advocates to promote, normalize and otherwise advocate for breastfeeding. Lactivists engage in a variety of activities that use biology and scientific research to create new identities and socialities. Lee (2018a), Falls (2017) and Wilson (2018) describe how breastfeeding and breastfeeding advocacy facilitate the emergence of new forms of identity and sociality. Robyn Lee argues for breastfeeding as a *poiesis* or 'art-of-living', which constrains but also allows for new possibilities in how we understand embodiment, care and kinship (2018a: 11). For Falls, lactivism is implicit in milk sharing, and the sociality it creates appears as a 'heterarchical counternetwork' that creates a form of 'free space', a new ground 'of experience, new modes of reason and freedom, and an instrument of critical transformation" (2017:198). Likewise, Wilson (2018) describes exceptional breastfeeding as the beginning of a movement. There are strong parallels between Lee's *poiesis*, Falls' free space, and Wilson's exceptional breastfeeding with the biological citizenship's hopeful model of democratization, agency and transformative action.

In contrast, in her book *Militant Lactivism? Attachment Parenting and Intensive Motherhood in the UK and France*, Charlotte Faircloth (2013), while noting that lactivism constitutes a form of identity work (and that science and scientific knowledge constitute part of this work), argues that lactivism places extreme demands of 'embodied maternal labour' (p 137) on women. While Faircloth does not explicitly engage with biological citizenship as a theoretical framework to analyze attachment parenting, her observation that lactivism simultaneously empowers women while demanding extreme embodied, financial and personal sacrifice speaks to the ways biopower is operationalized in misogynistic, patriarchal ways.

As we demonstrate in the coming chapters, our analysis of milk-sharing practices could trouble notions of milk sharing as biological citizenship. Specifically, our participants do not always (or even frequently) describe their activities as activist. For many milk-sharing participants, sharing milk is a way for mothers to meet AAP and WHO recommendations to exclusively breastfeed. In this sense, they are accepting and adhering – even hyper-adhering – to state mandates to breastfeed. Thus, while milk sharing seems to elicit new forms of identity making and biosociality, the biological citizenship framework may be limited for understanding milk sharers. This may be in part because it does not engage with a central characteristic of milk sharing that makes it different from other biological causes that bring people together: milk sharing is inherently interembodied and intimate.

In her book *Others' Milk*, Wilson (2018) proposes the notion of 'intimate citizenship' as one way of understanding exceptional breastfeeding.[5] Originally proposed by Ken Plummer (1993), intimate citizenship describes the blurring of boundaries between private decisions and public dialogue. It represents a bridge between the personal and the political. Building on Plummer's framework, Lisa Smyth (2008) argues that breastfeeding is a site of intimate citizenship because it brings together public policies that support breastfeeding for the health of the population and breastfeeding as a private decision and often private practice. Plummer's (1993) conceptualization of citizenship, loosely defined as a form of belonging to a collectivity, is similar to the notion of citizenship underlying Rose and Novas' (2005) biological citizenship. However, intimate citizenship deals with questions of what is considered private or public, and Wilson (2018) expands the notion to consider how milk sharing (and other forms of exceptional breastfeeding) might bring caregivers together in solidarity as something that simultaneously brings emotional satisfaction and constitutes moral action. Thus, while biological citizenship may address how milk sharing brings people together through a joint biological experience, intimate citizenship touches on the ways milk sharing blurs the boundaries between what is typically considered private behavior, caregivers' feeding choices and practices, and public action – the giving and taking of human milk through semipublic social networks as well as the myriad public responses to the practice.

Biological citizenship helps us elucidate the relationship between the emergence of community and the biological nature of lactation and infant feeding, and intimate citizenship accounts for the ways the practice violates traditional views of bodily boundedness. Both frameworks, with their foci on socialities produced by shared experiences and goals, are also highly compatible with the communities of practice framework. However, neither framework considers how the materiality of human milk and the labour involved in its production may affect the particular communities that emerge through milk sharing.

Bio-intimacy

Rhonda Shaw (Shaw and Morgan 2017; Shaw 2019) notes that peer milk sharing creates networks of bio-intimacy. Bio-intimacy, a concept advanced by Kroløkke and Peterson (2017) in their analysis of discourses surrounding uterine transplants and commercial surrogacy in Sweden and Denmark, builds on Lauren Berlant's (2008) view of intimacy as 'some sort of *genre*, involving hegemonic scripts that circulate in the public sphere and migrate to the private as a feeling of belonging' (Kroløkke and Peterson 2017: 193,). This view contrasts with common perceptions of intimacy as privately held feelings of closeness that are independent of social norms, thereby illuminating the 'feeling rules' (Hochschild 1983) that govern emotions and relations even in the private sphere. According to this view of intimacy, dominant societal scripts normalize certain relations as intimate, such as heterosexuality and a desire for a traditional nuclear family with biological offspring, while making others, such as same-sex relations and commercial reproduction, appear void of intimacy. Thus, societal definitions of intimacy affect internal feelings of connectedness and create patterns of belonging (Kroløkke and Peterson 2017).

Bio-intimacy encompasses the socially defined relationships and connectedness that are entangled in the sharing of biological material and human vitality, which are continually being reconfigured with new advances in biotechnology. Charlotte Kroløkke and Michael Peterson argue that reproductive technologies such as uterine transfer and surrogacy 'are technologies that re-enact the ability to create an intimate other – an "own" baby' (2017: 193). While these biotechnologies have the potential to create new social relationships, they 'build their legitimacy by drawing upon existing recognizable familial bio-intimate relations, affects, reproductive intent, and medical achievements' (2017: 193). Thus, these technologies are popular because they provide avenues for individuals who experience difficulty reproducing – due to infertility, uterine cancer, or same-sex partnership – to achieve bio-intimate relations that are socially defined as normative. How these relations are achieved, and the socially defined connectedness to others who make the relations possible – uterine donors, surrogates and so on – is shaped by broader cultural meanings and discourse. That is, the relationship is not embedded in the biological material itself but instead is determined by hegemonic social scripts that are negotiated depending on circumstance. Discourses of altruism, typically understood as a practice of disinterested concern for the wellbeing of others (Comte 1974 [1855]; Wuthnow 1993), and gift giving, which we understand as the unremunerated exchange of an item from one person to another in the context of establishing or fulfilling a social obligation (Mauss 1950 [1925]; Strathern 1990), are utilized to construct commercial surrogacy as an ethical solution to fertility challenges, defining the surrogate as a helper rather than an intimate member of the family she helps create (Kroløkke and Peterson 2017). However, in cases of uterine transfer, which is more commonly enacted by a friend or family member and takes place without formal compensation, the donor is more often positioned in intimate proximity, as an 'extended' family member to the resulting child. Both instances reinforce the legitimacy of the nuclear family and instate the primacy of genetic connectedness between parent and child. Kroløkke and Peterson (2017) argue that these technologies provide new mechanisms for citizenship through reproduction.

Drawing on this conceptualization of bio-intimacy, Shaw (2019) analyzes how altruism and intimacy operate in the instances of live kidney donation and peer milk sharing. Shaw's analysis utilizes distinctions between 'hard' and 'soft' altruism, in which hard altruism is self-sacrificial, voluntary and non-reciprocal, whereas soft altruism involves reciprocation. Anonymous, non-directed live kidney donation involves altruistic giving, no reciprocation, and anonymity, thereby falling closer to the 'hard' altruism end of the spectrum. However, cultural scripts that guide this form of kidney donation prioritize reason over emotion, defining altruism as a questionable motivation for donating. Institutions that control kidney donation have been known to reject potential anonymous, non-directed donors who provide altruistic reasons for wanting to donate, instead requiring them to provide rational motivations, such as describing a kidney as an excess organ, or awareness of the pain and suffering of individuals who are in need. Shaw argues that these cultural scripts align 'with Peter Singer's (2015) definition of "effective altruism" based on the careful calculation of "the most good [a person] can do" rather than being rooted in emotion and empathy. In this normative account, the prospective donor does not "feel" altruism, they do it, eschewing personal gain and ties to others' (2019: 561).

In contrast, Shaw (2019) argues that peer milk sharing is driven by 'affective altruism', where individuals' reasons for giving are rooted in emotion and empathy for another. This form of giving is more in line with 'soft' altruism because it is reciprocal, not anonymous, and creates a shared sense of belonging. Although monetary compensation is typically taboo in peer milk sharing, donors may experience reciprocation for their donations in the forms of community relationships, a sense of collective effort and commitment to feeding breastmilk to babies, and elevated identities as moral citizens (Shaw and Morgan 2017; Reyes-Foster and Carter 2018a, 2018b; Shaw 2019). Shaw posits the following:

> In the process of donating excess or surplus breastmilk for others to consume, breastmilk donors and peer milk sharers construct networks of bio-intimacy through which they forge relational and caring ties, as well as objectifying their moral identities with friend, family and community groups as generous and kind-hearted. In this respect, bio-intimate sharing of breastmilk is a form of biological citizenship that extends to a range of others beyond immediate family and friends with whom the donor shares a common project. (2019: 563)

Again, this framework is also evocative of communities of practice through its engagement in joint enterprise.

Emotional materiality

Theories of biological citizenship, intimate citizenship and bio-intimacy facilitate understanding of the sociality of human milk sharing, emphasizing the emergence of community bonds and relationships through the sharing of biological material. We build on these frameworks to account for the materiality of human milk and how this affects the operation of communities of practice. Susan Falls (2017) introduces a materialist analysis in her discussion of human milk sharing, arguing that human milk can be viewed as agentive because of its effects and interactions with other entities. The milk itself is as much an actor in the milk-sharing network as donors and recipients. To carry these analyses of peer milk sharing forward, we introduce the concept of emotional materiality, arguing that the emotional materiality of gifted milk allows its use as a generative conduit of bio-intimacy. We argue that this bio-intimacy becomes the foundation for bio-communities of practice.

Anna's story, which opens this chapter, exemplifies many of the struggles encountered by parents who seek milk. As we can see, her journey was not easy: in order to provide Grace with donor milk, Anna spent significant emotional resources, time and effort to secure what she believed was the best possible nutrition for her baby. When she says that a full freezer of milk is "like Christmas", or she describes the great lengths to which she will go to prevent any waste at all, she evokes what we call the emotional materiality of human milk. In this section, we develop the concept of emotional materiality, which, through its connection to Marxist materialism (Marx 1967 [1867]), inherently relates to labour and value. We argue that the emotional materiality of milk is constituted through the labour – emotional and material – involved in producing and obtaining it.

Because of this, shared milk resists commodification despite the labour involved in its production. Our research echoes the findings of Susan Falls, Kristin Wilson and others who have studied milk sharing in the Global North (Shaw 2007, 2015, 2019; Cassidy 2012a, 2012b; Thorley 2012; Gribble 2013, 2018; Palmquist and Doehler 2014, 2016; Stuebe et al 2014; Palmquist 2015; Falls 2017; Wilson 2018): sharing is seen by our research community as antithetical to selling. As we learned more about the motivations and experiences of women who give and receive human milk, we saw that milk sharing in the forms we were observing resisted other kinds of materialist analyses centred on commodification and alienation. This led us to ask what it is about human milk that makes sharing it so special. As we describe in this book, milk makes a priceless gift but a worthless commodity to the people we worked with in milk-sharing communities. However, it is important to note the intersectional privilege inherent in this notion: not all who share their milk are able to do so without compensation. Additionally, the history of the exploitation of Black women's reproductive bodies may contribute to alternate forms of infant feeding among Black women (Blum 1999; A Negro Nurse 2001; Shaw 2007; Harrison 2016). Shonda, a Black International Board Certified Lactation Consultant (IBCLC) who runs one of the largest breastfeeding support communities in Central Florida, attributed low milk sharing in the local Black community to 'Post Traumatic Slave Syndrome' – the historical memory of Black enslaved women who were forced to nurse their owners' babies at the expense of their own. This perspective is echoed in Wilson's (2018) discussion of milk sharing in Black communities. At the heart of this juxtaposition is a question of *value*, and value is inextricably intertwined with labour, as we explore in the following section.

Milk and value

Falls (2017) notes the importance of considering the value of milk in understanding its circulation in society. In her discussion, she draws a parallel between how gold and human milk are valued. Like gold, milk is cherished and desired. However, the primary difference is that while the value of gold has long been tied to other sociopolitical and economic concerns, milk has historically been valued insofar as it was a guarantee of life, and the fact that it was necessarily tied to a female body introduces further nuance: when commodified, wet nursing was frequently undervalued, and wet nurses were resented for the fact that their existence was necessary for the creation of this vital, life-sustaining nutrient. As gender scholars have noted, women's 'leaky bodies' have long been devalued and observed with suspicion (Longhurst 2001; Carter 2010; Shildrick 2015; Van Amsterdam 2015). The creation of infant formula, which eventually resulted in the disappearance of wet nurses, and concomitantly, the plunging of breastfeeding rates, is the ultimate erasure of the required feminine bodily presence for infant survival. The resurgence of breastfeeding in the US is often traced back to the devout group of Catholic women who founded La Leche League in the 1950s and published *The Womanly Art of Breastfeeding*. Breastfeeding was subsequently embraced by the natural childbirth movement in the 1960s and 1970s (Mathews and Zadak 1991; Golden 1996; Blum 1999). In the late 20th and 21st centuries, research developments on the science of human milk has resulted in the revaluing of breastmilk as a substance that simply cannot be replicated through scientific means. But this revaluing is not a revaluing of breastfeeding; rather, it is a revaluing only of breastmilk itself. For instance, workplace policies meant to support breastfeeding actually only support breastmilk pumping, as paid parental leave remains elusive in the US (Boswell-Penc and Boyer 2007; Johnson and Salpini 2017; Porter 2018; Johnson 2019).

If it is breastmilk that is valued, not breastfeeding, we can see that women continue to be erased from infant feeding. This is the crux of feminist social scientists' critiques of pumping, that the emergence of this technology has resulted in the separation of milk from the bodies of mothers, marking a first step in its transformation into a commodity (Van Esterik 1989, 1996; Stearns 2010; Ryan et al 2013; Team and Ryan 2014). However, by deploying this technology to harness excess milk, save it, and gift it, donors change the stakes: donors may value their milk because of the labour involved in extracting it, and because of the power their milk holds to transform not only their own babies' bodies, but those of other people's babies. Making milk becomes a superpower, giving milk becomes hero work. As we describe in this book, donors, rather than feeling disempowered or disconnected from their own milk, embrace the value generated through the work of pumping, collecting, storing and gifting. Recipients, desperately seeking to give their babies the best nutrition possible, cherish the gifts obtained after hours of internet searching, communicating with and screening potential donors, and driving long distances.

Biovalue and the gift

In order to understand how shared milk is imbued with value, one possibility is to consider the way in which value has been theorized in relation to other kinds of human products such as plasma, semen, or tissue. In her research on tissue economies, Catherine Waldby (2002) develops the notion of biovalue. Biovalue is created through technological processing. It encompasses laboratory processes that modify human tissues in order to increase their vitality. Thus, donated blood holds no value until it is turned into plasma through a series of technological transformations. Likewise, in settings where human milk has been institutionally commodified, raw donor milk is treated as a potentially harmful fluid. It is not until milk has been duly processed – homogenized, pasteurized, tested for bacteria and nutritional composition, rendered commercially sterile or turned into a human milk-based fortifier – that it is transformed from 'body dirt' into 'liquid gold' (Carroll 2014), becoming a valuable commodity.

In *Tissue Economies*, Waldby and Mitchell (2006) detail legal arguments about the nature of blood and tissue donation that have ultimately classified blood and tissues simultaneously as gifts and commodities. Considering the histories of blood and tissue banking, Waldby and Mitchell note that the legal definition of blood as gift rather than commodity was linked to an argument of scientific progress.[6] Waldby and Mitchell argue that institutions of tissue exchange embraced the rhetoric of the gift as a way of divesting 'donors' of property rights over their blood, tissues and other bodily products, paving the way for the commodification of body products such as stem lines. Alongside Waldby and Mitchell's work on tissue economies, Kara Swanson's (2011, 2014) social history of body banking, particularly the banking of blood, milk and semen, considers the ways in which the very notion of 'banking' is central to the commodification of human body products. The language of banking, Swanson argues, 'straitjackets' the use of human body parts and in turn reproduces inequalities in medical care. This is because the language of banking is inextricably tied to the US neoliberal medical industry, which is inherently market- and profit-driven. Body banking, even non-profit human milk banking, and biovalue represent two sides of the same neoliberal coin. Although Swanson and Waldby and Mitchell are not in explicit conversation with one another, there are strong areas of commonality between Waldby and Mitchell's argument about biovalue and Swanson's analysis of body banking, as both explore the transformation of body products into commodities.

The logics of biovalue underlying banked milk are evident in the way the technological processing, donor-screening and testing processes are emphasized in both non-profit banking and bioventure capitalism. Milk is not considered fully safe until it is processed. The processing of human milk in the context of the milk bank severs the relationship between the donor and recipient, and transforms milk from food to medicine (Shaw 2010; Zizzo 2011; Landers and Hartmann 2013; Carroll 2014, 2015; Carroll et al 2014; Shaw and Morgan 2017). The use of processed milk in medical settings is emphasized as for-profit ventures such as Medolac Laboratories and Prolacta Bioscience explicitly position themselves in competition with non-profit, HMBANA-affiliated milk banks. However, all of these companies appeal to a moral sensibility: Medolac explicitly markets itself as a 'public benefit' corporation, and HMBANA milk banks put their non-profit status front and centre, recognizing the inherent 'goodness' of human milk (Hassan 2010; Harrison 2019). This appeal to morality and 'doing good' is also identified in the context of other forms of bodily donation, including blood, organs and reproductive surrogacy (Titmuss 1997; Waldby 2002; Rudrappa and Collins 2015; Hovav 2019; Shaw 2019).

In the late 1960s, when blood transfusions were primarily of whole (relatively unprocessed) blood, Titmuss (1997) theorized blood donation as a form of intercorporeality and 'civil intersubjectivity'. Waldby and Mitchell (2006) point out that as the processes for donating and using blood and human tissues have changed over time, so too has the way the tissue economy has been understood. As blood 'became more mobile, flexible, and specialized', it also became 'a global commodity brokered by international pharmaceutical companies' (Waldby and Mitchell 2006: 49). Although blood donation discourses still contain appeals to good citizenship and altruism, the commodification of blood resulting from technological innovations has also resulted in the regular practice of compensated plasma donation. Like blood, human milk is a renewable resource, albeit a temporary one. Like blood, milk undergoes a series of transformations as it is processed in both the banking and bioventure capitalist contexts (Swanson 2011, 2014).

However, peer-shared milk entirely circumvents the laboratory. Even the non-profit organization Get Pumped, which provides a 'semi-formal' model, does not process the milk it distributes. In this way, peer milk sharing is closer to the 'whole blood' donation of the early and mid-20th century or even organ donation than it is to contemporary body banking. In contrast to plasma recipients, organ transplant patients describe the tissue economy of organ donation as highly personal, describing the feeling that part of the donor's 'self or personhood has been transmitted along with the organ' (Fox and Swazey 1992: 36). This notion is echoed in older discourses of wet nursing, often expressed as concerns that wet nurses' dubious character may be transmitted to the nurslings they fed (Sussman 1982; Wolf 1999; Reyes-Foster and Carter 2018a). In our research and other studies of milk sharing, peer milk donors often expressed the satisfaction derived from watching babies grow and thrive on their milk. They, too, describe milk donation as highly personal. Because it is characterized by the direct gifting of unprocessed milk from one person to another and *not* constituted through technological processing, peer-shared milk does not have biovalue. It is possible that this – the fact that shared milk is not tied to biovalue – is why we encounter such resistance to commodification in milk-sharing communities. However, on recognition that shared milk does not have biovalue, we also recognize that it is still valued in an inherently unique way, one that is tied to a different process. We call this value, imbued in milk through labour and affect, 'emotive value'.

Emotive value

Despite the fact that, through its separation from the human body, milk becomes a commodity, monetary value appears to instill milk with suspicion (Golden 1996; Boyer 2010; Shaw 2019). In this sense, human milk appears to mimic Durkheim's (1947 [1912]) classic dichotomy of the sacred and profane: human milk is sacred, its value irreducible to monetary worth. Yet, when a profit motive is introduced, the sacred object is contaminated and becomes profane. As a sacred object, we might even call human milk, frozen in bags and treasured in women's freezers, a fetish. While Marx (1967 [1867]) wrote of commodity fetishism as a feature of capitalism, a drive to possess as many commodities as possible, human milk as fetish harkens back to an older definition: originally, 'fetish' described objects believed to contain magical qualities. The materiality of the fetish is what made the concept so appealing to Marx – in commodity fetishism, it is the accumulation of these objects that drives capitalist markets (Marx 1967 [1867]). Similarly, possessing human milk brings joy and relief to milk recipients – when they see their freezers full of milk, they know their babies' food source is guaranteed, and they marvel at the physical effect this milk has on their infants as they grow and thrive on donor milk. Grateful recipients proudly and happily post pictures of happy, chunky babies smiling, surrounded by bags of frozen milk, in online social media. Others create beautiful collages of their babies with pictures of their donors' babies, writing of the milk siblings who have generously shared their mothers' milk.

For recipient mothers, the milk in their freezers has the ability to bestow on their children the benefits of breastfeeding even as they themselves are unable to exclusively breastfeed. I (Beatriz) remember the disproportionate joy I experienced the first time my baby's stool returned to a mustard-yellow colour and smelled of breastmilk after it had turned green, fetid and pasty when his demand outpaced my supply and I resorted to formula feeding. Being able to give Rowan only breastmilk motivated me to continue to breastfeed him, and our breastfeeding relationship continued until he was nearly three years old. My experience reflects the findings of Aunchalee Palmquist and Kirsten Doehler (2016), who found that mothers who used shared milk tended to continue breastfeeding beyond the AAP-recommended first year of life and more in line with the WHO recommendation of at least two years or as long as mother and infant feel comfortable. Another recent study found that, among mothers with low milk supply, those who supplemented with peer-shared milk breastfed longer than those who supplemented with formula (Cassar-Uhl and Liberatos 2018). Seeing rolls of fat appear on my son's thighs almost overnight when weeks before his weight gain had slowed precipitously felt magical even when I knew, logically, that the reason he was gaining weight was because he was ingesting more calories, and he likely would have gained weight if I had chosen to give him formula. Yet, I experienced a deep emotional satisfaction derived from knowing that my baby was on an all-human milk diet and felt anguished whenever I gave him a bottle of formula. Remembering this emotional turmoil helped me better understand the way that many of our recipient parents spoke about using gifted milk. In describing her experiences of using banked donor milk for her children, Wilson also notes that the decision was primarily emotional:

> I was able to get the milk for my children with prescriptions from compliant doctors and all of my savings. Emotions guided my decision to give my sons breastmilk … I should try to give my children any kind of head start I could, even if the science backing breastmilk was unclear and the cost was astronomical. My sons would have fared just fine on formula. (2018: 231)

The relationship that milk sharers have with milk, whether they gift it or receive it, contains important emotional dimensions (Cassidy and

El Tom 2010; Thorley 2014; Falls 2017; Shaw and Morgan 2017; Gribble 2018; Shafer et al 2018; Wilson 2018; Lee 2019; McCloskey and Karandikar 2019; Shaw 2019). The gift of human milk contains within it this emotional materiality.

Marilyn Strathern (1990) notes that gifts are inalienable because they are repositories of relationships. The extensive labour required in regularly donating and receiving milk from others takes place within a moral gift economy. Donors see themselves as contributing to a greater good, enacting intimate and biological citizenship (Shaw and Morgan 2017; Shaw 2019). This labour imbues human milk with the form of value we call emotive value. Emotive value thus accounts for the emotional materiality of gifted human milk. Like people in other milk-sharing communities (Thorley 2012; Gribble 2014b, 2018; Palmquist 2015; Falls 2017; Wilson 2018), mothers in the milk-sharing communities we studied care where their milk goes and where it comes from. Unlike monetary value or even biovalue, the emotive value that imbues milk is connected to broader questions of mothering, community and beliefs about doing good in the world: the emotive value of shared milk is constituted through the labour involved in its expression, storage, transportation, exchange and handling, the relationships it helps develop, and the mutual prioritization of infant health among donors and recipients. Beyond building a community or feeding hungry babies, it is milk itself, as a physical, biological, material substance, that elicits these connections. This fact warrants an examination of the role milk plays as a material actor in peer milk sharing.

The vibrancy of milk

Milk is material. It flows from mammal bodies into bottles and storage bags. It fills freezers and infants' stomachs. Most importantly, milk makes babies grow, turning tiny newborns into cherub-like babies and babbling toddlers. In recent years, scholars have turned their attention to questions of ontology – that is, the question of being. An ontological approach seeks to address some of the shortcomings of social constructionism, particularly by trying to address material realities for humans and non-humans alike. In ontological, materialist approaches, matter is generative, vibrant and active. 'What would happen to our thinking about politics', writes Jane Bennett, 'if we took more seriously the idea that natural and technological materialities were themselves actors alongside and within us?' (Bennett 2010: 46). These ideas are also visible in the work of anthropologist Arjun Appadurai, whose notion of things in motion recognizes that objects move in and out of various states as part of their 'career'. For Appadurai, objects are not static entities but 'one phase in the life of some things' (1986: 17).

Our approach considers the materiality of milk itself and the ways this materiality is tied to value. In this sense, milk sharing, based almost entirely on human bodies' ability (or inability) to lactate and humans' freedom to choose to gift and seek out gifted milk can be read as an exercise in feminist freedom (Gaard 2013; Carter and Reyes-Foster 2017; Falls 2017; Wilson 2018). As Wilson (2018) demonstrates, this exercise in feminist freedom expands rather than limits possibilities for reproductive inclusion for individuals who are transgender or gender non-binary, acknowledging lactation as gendered practice but expanding traditional notions of which gendered bodies are allowed to participate.

Beyond an exercise in freedom, a materialist analysis can be used to study milk as an actor capable of agency. Most useful for such an analysis is Jane Bennett's writing on the agency of objects, particularly of edible matter. In *Vibrant Matter*, Bennett (2010) describes objects as 'actants', capable of agency in the world. Eating, writes Bennett, constitutes a series of transformations between human and non-human bodies. As David Goodman points out, food is an 'ontologically real and active, lively presence' (2001: 183).[7]

In this framework, what makes human milk active and lively is physical: it is the only biological substance that exists solely for the sustenance of human infants. Its biological qualities, which include particular biomarkers, bacteria, immune factors, and a nutritional composition uniquely tailored to an infant's age (Hinde and Milligan 2011; Quinn et al 2012, 2016; Miller 2015), are incomparable to human milk substitutes or other foods. Thus, while artificial infant milks may adequately nourish any child, the exact biological processes by which human milk is consumed and digested by human infants is still in the process of being understood. This is not a question of whether 'breast is best' or even superior to infant formulas. Simply put, scientific understanding of the biological and biocultural processes of breastfeeding is incipient, but this early research suggests that the production and feeding of human milk is more complex than previously imagined (Tomori et al 2016; Quinn 2018). Breastmilk is qualitatively different from artificial infant milk: where formula is inert, human milk is teeming with life.

As Bennett (2010) explains, the effect of food on bodies can only be understood as a non-linear system. Human milk is an assemblage of living elements that in turn interact within a growing infant body. In the 19th century, many philosophers 'believed that food had the power to shape the dispositions of people and nations' (Bennett 2010: 43). Thus, foods were understood to contain qualities –moral, energetic, vital – that would then be transmitted to those who consumed them. During this same time period, breastmilk was not only believed to nourish newborns, but also to pass on moral character, and physicians expressed concern that wet nurses could pass on strange humours to the infants they fed (Sussman 1982).

If we accept Bennett's (2010) argument that all matter is vibrant, it is easy to conceptualize the inherent vibrancy of human milk. In saying this, we are not being anthropocentric and suggesting that this applies only to humans, but instead we mean there is inherent vibrancy in all mammals' milks as they exist to nourish the young of their specific species. In this sense, the vibrancy of human milk is specific to humans in the same way that whale milk would be specific to whales. Although humans and animals can and do engage in interspecies milk consumption, our interest is in exploring the relationship between the inherent and unique vibrancy of human milk as it pertains to human milk sharing. In some hyper-individualist discourses, human milk is portrayed as highly individuated. To a certain extent, this is true; that is, each individual human's milk is 'custom-made' for one particular baby. The baby is believed to communicate its needs through signaling biomarkers (called the 'baby backwash' theory), stimulating the mother to produce exactly the milk the baby needs (Al-Shehri et al 2015; Breakey et al 2015; Hinde 2016). The mother's own milk also contains what she consumes, sometimes necessitating that she eliminate certain foods (dairy, gluten, broccoli) when the baby shows a sensitivity to it. In the milk-bank context, milk is analyzed for nutritional composition because premature and medically fragile babies need more nutritionally dense milk, which is produced by mothers of younger babies. Nevertheless, a donor's milk will nourish any recipient baby, and that baby – barring any sensitivity to the mothers' diet, or a rejection on the basis of taste such as in the case of high-lipase milk, or an underlying health problem – will thrive on that milk.

In peer milk sharing, participants connect with each other and the milk itself in deeply emotional ways (Cassidy and El Tom 2010; Gribble 2014b, 2014c, 2018; Thorley 2014; Falls 2017; Shaw and Morgan 2017; Shafer et al 2018; Wilson 2018; Lee 2019; McCloskey and Karandikar 2019; Shaw 2019). We call this connection between emotive value and materiality the 'emotional materiality of milk'. The emotional materiality of milk is the foundation of bio-communities of practice. While milk is attributed social meaning, it is also a living, vital substance that directly contributes to the way humans use and grow from it.

Bio-communities of practice

If milk-sharing communities of practice are sites for the production of bio-intimacy created through the exchange of human milk, we can conceptualize these communities as bio-communities of practice. In contrast to communities of practice that can exist for any reason or shared goal, bio-communities of practice are constituted through bio-intimacy. Without it, the trust and affective connections that are created through the sharing of biological material would not be possible. By the same token, these bio-communities of practice retain the social learning aspect of communities of practice. Bio-intimacy is established as participants learn the processes involved and the spoken and unspoken norms surrounding membership in these communities, and they reproduce it by sharing images and information online and through face-to-face interactions.

Whereas in biological citizenship individuals see themselves as sharing a joint sense of belonging through a biological category and jointly taking a stake in the society at large (Rose and Novas 2005), bio-communities of practice are primarily concerned with establishing networks on a smaller scale. In biological citizenship, members often come together to advocate for legal recognition or rights from the state (Rose and Novas 2005). Bio-communities of practice are not necessarily engaged in political advocacy work. Instead, the focus of the group is facilitating the availability of human milk to babies who need it, and in so doing, they establish bio-intimate, affective relationships (Shaw and Morgan 2017; Shaw 2019). Bio-communities of practice may facilitate biological citizenship through breastfeeding activism and promotion, although we posit that the two are conceptually distinct.

A key characteristic of bio-communities of practice is the self-generating nature of the group. Without participants willing to donate and receive milk, the community disappears. The goals of the bio-communities of practice are immediate rather than long term. Participants focus on creating and distributing breastmilk in the here and now. There is inherent turnover in membership. As the goals of the group no longer become relevant to some individuals' lives, new individuals find themselves in situations that bring them into the communities. Central participants – those who are experienced, committed, or more heavily invested – socialize new participants, who may become central over time or may remain peripheral, participating only on occasion. In this sense, the group is generative. While a shared goal of feeding babies human milk remains present, members engage in the work to achieve their goals themselves rather than advocating for assistance from the outside.

Examination of central and peripheral participants, their relationships to one another, and their milk-sharing practices facilitates analysis of how power and social inequalities operate within peer milk sharing bio-communities of practice. In her analysis of peer breastmilk sharing in southeastern Georgia, US, Falls conceptualizes the milk-sharing networks in which she was an observer and participant as a 'heterarchy', defined as 'a form of social organization that is flexible and adaptive, in which relationships shift with context, and where power is contextual' (2017: 21). In a heterarchy, individuals' relationships may be complex, but they are not positioned within a hierarchy. Falls views milk-sharing networks as heterarchical because donors and recipients are co-constitutive, meaning one cannot exist without the other. Participants can take on various roles, shifting from donor to recipient, or becoming a moderator of a Facebook group that facilitates milk sharing, such as Human Milk 4 Human Babies or Eats on Feets. These relationships are heterarchical because they resist the overt power differential present in common organizational and institutional arrangements, such as education institutions (teacher to student), business (supervisor to worker) and government (police officer to citizen).

The communities of practice model suggests that although strict hierarchical arrangements may be absent, expert-to-apprentice relationships are central to transferring knowledge and continuation of practices (Soden and Halliday 2000). This is also the case in bio-communities of practice. Novice, or peripheral, participants are often introduced to milk sharing and learn how it takes place from central ('expert') participants who have engaged in the practices longer or more frequently, or who have specialized knowledge through their professional or organizational engagement. From a communities of practice perspective, these relationships are fundamentally power relationships. Wenger writes:

> The definition of the regime of accountability and of who gets to qualify as competent are questions of power. Every learning move is a claim to competence which may or may not function – i.e., be considered legitimate by the community or change the criteria for competence that the community has developed.... Learning and power imply each other. (2010: 188)

Thus, power dynamics are inherent to communities of practice (and, consequently, bio-communities of practice as well), but they are not predetermined or fixed. Wenger continues: 'The accountability and identification that form the basis for power in communities is horizontal, mutual, negotiated, often tacit and informal' (2010: 189).

The overall lack of diversity based on race and class in our study and others on milk sharing limits our ability to fully assess how social inequalities operate within these networks (Paynter and Goldberg 2018), although some forms of inequality have been identified. In a quantitative analysis of the characteristics of parents who participate in online milk sharing in the US, Palmquist and Doehler (2014) found that milk-sharing participants were largely white, middle-class women, with donors having a slight yet significant income and education advantage over recipients. Whether or not such inequalities, which carry significance within broader society, affect the relationships within peer milk-sharing communities is unclear. Although disparities are found between donors and recipients, recipients remain able to provide exclusive breastmilk to their babies through their relationships with donors and their mutual engagement in milk sharing (Palmquist and Doehler 2014). Wenger (2010) explains that the power imbued in an individual's status as an 'expert' within a community of practice is not likely to translate to greater power or higher social status outside the group. Likewise, it may also be the case that occupying a social position that is imbued with more power in society may not correspond with greater power within a community of practice. Wilson (2018) found that the milk-sharing participants she studied reached across often-divisive social categories such as religion and political affiliation to fulfill the more immediate purpose of feeding human milk. In her study, the divisions and power inequalities identified in the broader society did not seem to affect who would share milk with whom.

However, milk-sharing participants and researchers observe other forms of hierarchy within milk-sharing communities. Studies reveal 'hierarchies of need', where some potential recipients are viewed as needier than others, and are thus often prioritized by donors (Gribble 2014b; Falls 2017; Wilson 2018). Those who are perceived as being at the top of the hierarchy – babies who are adopted, whose mothers are ill or deceased, or who are ill themselves – are more likely to be prioritized by donors, and are more able to acquire milk than those who fall lower in the hierarchy of need. Recipient mothers who are perceived as not conforming to societal standards of 'moral motherhood' may be identified as unworthy recipients, and therefore be denied access to peer milk (Shaw and Morgan 2017; Reyes-Foster and Carter 2018a, 2018b).

These insights show that although milk sharers may come together to form more-or-less egalitarian associations, their interconnections are not fully void of power inequalities. At the same time, as a community of practice, power is not distributed systematically through a strict and unwavering hierarchy. Instead, it is enacted and negotiated through the ongoing practices and meanings generated within the group, and in the relationships among and between central and peripheral participants, whose positions within the group are also variable (Lave and Wenger 1991).

Although this research focuses on milk sharing, other social practices may also be conceptualized within the bio-communities of practice framework. For example, this framework may be useful for examining other forms of shared reproductive labor, such as surrogacy or sperm donation. Laura Mamo (2007) describes practices used by some lesbian couples to inseminate by obtaining sperm by known and trusted donors. Some of her participants developed informal community networks that helped lesbian couples identify gay men who were willing to give their sperm to assist in family formation. The relationships between known sperm donors, lesbian parents, and the children conceived are negotiated, resulting a "complex web of interpersonal relationships" (Côté and Lavoie 2019: 165). These and other similar networks might constitute bio-communities of practice. As such, they hold promise for new forms of biological citizenship, thereby expanding kinship, belonging, and social and biological inclusion.

3

Entering Bio-Communities of Practice

Shannon and Beatriz first met at a coffee shop on campus during the beginning of the fall semester in 2013. I (Beatriz) was at the tail end of the first trimester of pregnancy with my second child. Unlike Shannon, I struggled, and ultimately was unable, to exclusively breastfeed my children. My first son, born as I was working to finish my dissertation, spent his first few days in the NICU, and I always believed that my inability to exclusively breastfeed him despite an environment that was generally supportive of breastfeeding was due to the fact that we were separated for the first few days of his life. My second child, another boy, was born under ideal circumstances. His birth was not traumatic, and we were able to initiate nursing immediately. The fact that I was now employed as a professor made the financial transition from one to two children fairly uneventful, and the flexibility of my schedule allowed me to spend most of my time with my baby, even when I returned to work (he became known as 'my appendage' because he spent most of his time in a wrap, sleeping against my chest). Nevertheless, his weight gain was extremely slow and his paediatrician became concerned. At his four-month appointment, my baby's weight had barely crept up from our prior checkup. On the growth charts, his weight had plummeted from the 24th percentile to the fifth.

Despite a parade of lactation consultants, breastfeeding support groups, 'power pumping' (aggressively pumping at short intervals to stimulate milk production), 'breastfeeding vacations' (stopping all activity and spending entire weekends in bed skin-to-skin with my baby), and an endless supply of various galactagogues (fenugreek, blessed thistle, fennel, moringa root, oatmeal, flax, brewer's yeast and Domperidone),[1] my supply simply couldn't keep up with his demand. I had completely bought into the notion, freely circulating in my support circles, that low milk supply was due to social causes, that it was an artificial phenomenon resulting from aggressive formula marketing and ill-informed pediatricians following inaccurate growth charts based on the growth patterns of formula-fed babies. It was extremely difficult to accept that I could not exclusively feed my baby, particularly as I was studying milk sharing and frequenting local breastfeeding support groups. A few days after this distressing checkup, I attended a support group meeting where I found myself conducting the most authentic kind of participant observation. I lamented my struggles to feed my baby. One of the women there said, "Why don't you ask Jill? She just gave birth to her surrogate baby and she's donating all her milk."

Jill, whom I knew through her work with Get Pumped, had intended to donate her milk after the birth of her surrogate baby. She had been posting pictures on Facebook of her milk as she pumped it and it transitioned from thick, yellow colostrum to creamy, white milk. I logged on to the social media platform, took a breath, and sent her a message explaining my situation. She responded almost immediately: "I can set aside ten ounces a day for you. Just come pick it up." For the next six months, we supplemented breastfeeding with Jill's milk. Once a week, I would throw ice into the cooler I kept in my car, drive to her home, and pick up a grocery bag or two filled with frozen milk. My baby, whose skinny legs I had anxiously squeezed, seemed to transform before my eyes, becoming plump and rapidly returning to a stable place on the growth charts. When my paediatrician asked what I had done to increase my baby's weight, I explained he was receiving donor milk. "That's wonderful!," she exclaimed.

My baby was one of 20 babies who benefitted from Jill's generous gift of milk. In her blog post about her experiences donating milk after surrogacy, she explained that she had a hard time breastfeeding her own two children and pumping, and that donating her milk helped her overcome feelings of failure resulting from these struggles. She wrote:

> 'I got over and healed from my mommy guilt from my 2 previous breastfeeding flops and was able to help babies thrive. Babies who were in the same situation that my own children went though, babies who were adopted and born addicted to drugs making them formula intolerant, one of my nieces, and even one other surrogate baby. There are 20 different stories I could tell you about the babies I've helped over the last 6 months but I can tell you I feel whole again and that mommy guilt is gone.'

Jill's and my journeys into milk sharing are unique in some respects but similar in many ways to the stories of milk sharing Shannon and I collected over the years doing research on milk sharing. In this chapter, we explore the multiple pathways that bring donors and recipients into milk-sharing bio-communities of practice, and consider the different motivations, practices and experiences of parents and caregivers who participate in the practice. Before discussing these pathways, we provide a brief snapshot of what the communities look like that potential participants are entering.

A multiplicity of bio-communities

In conceptualizing milk-sharing communities, we initially thought of the (singular) concept '*bio-community* of practice'. However, we found the term to be too limiting for describing the people and practices we observed. Whereas the concept of bio-community connotes a self-contained, homogenous, singular entity, the plural bio-communities is open-ended, multiple and heterogeneous. We observed that people who engaged in milk sharing did so in environments that fostered a variety of connections and practices. Moreover, people in our milk-sharing communities often belonged to several different social networks that sometimes, but not always, overlapped. For instance, a donor looking to make room in her freezer may be referred to a recipient by a local maternity care provider or by a member of a local Facebook group, or even by a mutual friend. These localized relationships take place within several broader, overlapping networks, some of which are organized by geographic location, and others which are not. Participants who lived closer to the coast had their own private online communities separate from those in Orlando, although Orlando's proximity to the coast meant that many participants were members of both. Dr Leila, a chiropractor who was known for her expertise working with pregnant women, newborns and children, practised in a smaller town between several different communities, saw patients from the city of Orlando as well as those in the surrounding suburbs, rural areas, and beach towns, and therefore often connected people from a variety of different groups. Peer milk sharing most often takes place at this level, where participants meet each other in person and know each other more intimately than they would through exclusive online interaction (Falls 2017; Palmquist and Doehler 2016; Reyes-Foster et al 2015, 2017; Thorley 2012; Wilson 2018). Relationships of bio-intimacy are established when a donor and recipient meet in person and the donor's biological material is transferred from one person to another (Shaw 2019; Shaw and Morgan 2017). This bio-intimacy is reinforced through subsequent communication between donors and recipients, including sharing of baby photos and through expressions of gratitude and sometimes friendship.

In addition to localized bio-communities where participants might know each other both online and 'in real life', or at least share mutual acquaintances, milk-sharing participants also belong to broader online communities with which they interact in meaningful ways (Cassidy 2012a; Gribble 2014a, 2014b, 2014c; Palmquist and Doehler 2014, 2016; Perrin et al 2014; Falls 2017). This may be through participation in large online communities with thousands of members, where participants directly share advice and their own stories, or even, at times, find donors or recipients. For example, one such group, the closed Facebook group Dairy Queens, has over 50,000 members. The purpose of the group is breastfeeding support, not specifically milk sharing, but in discussing the range of breastfeeding practices, milk sharing frequently emerges as a topic of discussion. These online forums are places where interconnectedness between people who milk share are reinforced and their practice is validated. In that sense, such forums may function as spaces of recruitment, particularly for those who are unfamiliar with peer milk sharing.

Members of milk-sharing bio-communities of practice may also participate in promoting breastfeeding or milk sharing by engaging in 'lactivist' activities, making and sharing memes, news stories and their own personal experiences with their broader social networks in an effort to normalize the sharing of human milk (Cassidy 2012a; Falls 2017; Wilson 2018). Wilson (2018) explores milk sharing as lactivism in her analysis of exceptional breastfeeding. This engagement in public discourse moves milk sharing from private practice into the public sphere, raising awareness of milk sharing among those who may have been unaware of it. This may elicit both support and criticism, but for people who engage in producing and disseminating a pro-milk-sharing stance, this public engagement affirms their identities and their connection and belonging to milk-sharing bio-communities of practice.

Through engagement in the communities, networks and spaces described earlier, people who participate in milk-sharing bio-communities of practice develop a sense of belonging to something greater than oneself, of participating in a global, ancestral community (Falls 2017; Giles 2017; Shaw and Morgan 2017; Shaw 2019). Underlying the bio-communities of practice is bio-intimacy, which fosters relationships and connections between participants but also between participants and the idea of milk sharing as meaningful. The emotional materiality and inherent vitality of human milk make giving and receiving it an emotionally powerful act, and engagement with others who have participated in the practice and affirm it further fosters bio-intimacy. The result is a sense of deep emotional and biological connection to others who share milk, both past and present.

Becoming a donor

Studies of breastmilk donation in milk-banking and peer-sharing contexts identify breastmilk donors as primarily cisgender women who have given birth, produce more milk than they need, have been introduced in some way to milk sharing or banking, and are willing to participate (Thorley 2012; Gribble 2014b; Palmquist and Doehler 2014, 2016; Palmquist 2015; Reyes-Foster et al 2015; Perrin et al 2016; Falls 2017; Wilson 2018). Similar to past research, donors in our study were all exclusively breastfeeding their own babies at the time of donation, although some supplemented with formula very early on. They varied in the ways they learned about milk sharing, their levels of commitment to milk donation, the meanings they attributed to giving milk, and the extent of their involvement in the practice. They took on different roles in the communities, with some remaining on the periphery and others becoming central participants. They remained active in the communities for a period of their lives, with even most who became central participants eventually moving to the periphery as their children grew older and their breastfeeding years came to a close, being replaced by others coming into the practice.

The paths participants took to become peer breastmilk donors can be classified into the three broad categories of abundant milk, intending to give, and giving by request. Participants in the abundant milk category, which was most common among survey and interview participants, were breastfeeding mothers who created more milk than they needed for their own child, and sought breastmilk sharing as a way of putting their milk to good use. Participants in the intending to give category decided they wanted to give their breastmilk early on, often before their babies were even born, and subsequently worked to produce enough milk to donate. The giving by request category consisted of participants who were not intending to give their breastmilk at all, but encountered someone in their social network who needed milk, and decided to donate in response to this need.

Abundant milk

The most common pathway to becoming a peer breastmilk donor, occurring among just over half of donors in our study, was that mothers found themselves with abundant milk and did not want it to go to waste. Participants in this category developed successful breastfeeding relationships with their babies and were expressing milk that slowly started to build up in their freezers. Recognizing that they had excess, often described as freezers "overflowing with milk", they sought ways to put their milk to good use. Not wanting to waste milk is consistently identified as a primary motivator for mothers to donate to milk banks (Arnold and Borman 1996; Azema and Callahan 2003; Osbaldiston and Mingle 2007; de Alencar and Seidle 2009) and to peers (Gribble 2014b; Perrin et al 2016; Shaw 2019), so it is not surprising that this was common among our study participants. Many were initially uncertain about what they could do with their milk, and their quest to find a way to put their milk to good use led them to peer milk sharing.

Different experiences led to the production of excess milk. Some participants experienced oversupply, where they produced more milk than their babies needed. Oversupply can lead to breast engorgement, when the breasts become overfilled with milk, which can become painful and lead to other breastfeeding problems. Mothers in this category either expressed milk to relieve or avoid engorgement and promote comfort, or their expressed milk was originally intended for their own child. A few expressed milk because of breastfeeding difficulties or because their baby was sick or in the NICU.

Those who became donors due to abundant milk became either routine donors or occasional donors. Routine donors developed ongoing relationships with their recipients and worked to produce extra milk to give. They tended to eventually build a substantial milk supply or oversupply, although some experienced breastfeeding challenges early on. Becoming routine donors, they tended to donate high quantities of milk, totalling in the hundreds and thousands of ounces. Some donated all of their excess milk to one or two babies, whereas others had multiple recipients, such as Sara, who donated to more than 30 recipient babies. Routine donors in our study were central participants in milk-sharing bio-communities of practice because they maintained prolonged participation, shared comparatively large quantities of their biological material, became 'experts' in how peer milk is shared, and became emotionally invested in sharing milk. For occasional donors, giving milk was an infrequent or rare practice that simply allowed them to clear out an overflowing freezer. Participants who became occasional donors gained satisfaction from knowing their milk was going to good use and helping others, but they did not necessarily make extra sacrifices to ensure that they would have a regular supply of excess milk to give. Occasional donors were more likely to be peripheral participants in milk-sharing bio-communities of practice because they engaged only a few times, shared comparatively small quantities of their biological material, and often did not come to embody the situated knowledge, core values and emotional connectedness characteristic of central participants. However, some became more involved in peer milk sharing in other ways, such as moderating a milk-sharing group on Facebook, thereby becoming central participants to the practice while only donating their own milk on occasion.

Jane, the mother of two whom we introduced in Chapter 1, initially began milk sharing for the utilitarian purpose of not wasting her excess milk, and over time became a central participant in several peer milk-sharing communities. After exclusively breastfeeding her first child, Avery, she became a CLC and birth doula, establishing herself as a well-known figure in the natural birth and breastfeeding communities in the Orlando area. She became known among several birth professionals as someone who had excess milk, who would sometimes connect her with potential recipients. At the time of our interview, she had donated at least 2,000 ounces to about 12 direct recipients and to Get Pumped. She explained her entry into milk sharing:

> 'So initially, I was pretty much just pumping to keep my body comfortable. I would start feeling engorged and I would get uncomfortable so I would pump. So then, once I had a baby to pump for, I set up a pumping schedule and would pump a couple times a day. Because this baby needed my milk pretty much exclusively so I pumped pretty aggressively to keep up with her need.'

Like others who became routine donors, Jane became a milk donor as a way of utilizing the excess milk she produced. However, once she had a baby to donate to, she initiated a more rigorous pumping routine just to provide for her recipient baby. Thus, while her entry into peer milk sharing may be one of convenience and a desire to not waste her precious milk, she became a routine donor as a way of helping, and rearranged her life in significant ways to continue giving milk. This pattern, also identified in previous studies (Gribble 2013, 2014b; Falls 2017), illustrates how donors can move quickly from peripheral to central participants. As a result of her ongoing, weekly donations, Jane's recipient baby was able to meet the AAP recommendation of consuming exclusive breastmilk for the first six months of life.

Over the next few years, Jane found other recipients, and continued giving milk about once a week over the course of breastfeeding her two children into toddlerhood. Friends and birth professionals would tag her in Facebook posts made by mothers who were seeking milk, and Jane never turned anyone away. She had enough requests that she never posted on Facebook seeking recipients, and she never used Eats on Feets or Human Milk 4 Human Babies. This method of locating recipients through local networks was fairly typical of donors in our study: among donors who took our online survey, nearly 80% used the internet at some point to locate recipients, and while a majority used Eats on Feets or Human Milk 4 Human Babies at least once, about half also relied on local private Facebook groups and their own Facebook pages (Reyes-Foster et al 2015).

Jane usually gave her milk on a first-come, first-served basis, but occasionally she prioritized some recipients over others, enacting the 'hierarchies of need' identified in past research (Falls 2017; Wilson 2018). When asked if she did anything to screen recipients, she explained:

> 'No, if they need milk, they need milk. I have tended to, just this time, between Get Pumped and the other babies that have needed my milk, it's been newer babies or the baby that I'm donating to privately right now, she had some kind of surgery on her head. So, she really needs breastmilk. You know, supplementing with formula during the day would not be ideal for a baby that's recovering from intense surgery. But that's kind of the way it's fallen. I mean, I would have no problem donating to just anybody who just had low supply or anything but I seem to have been donating more to the high need babies this time.'

Later in the interview, Jane explained why she donated to Get Pumped rather than just directly to recipients:

> 'I do both. I chose to donate to Get Pumped specifically because they tend to get milk to the babies that the milk banks don't have enough milk for. They don't rank high enough on the priorities of the milk banks, but they aren't always these healthy normal babies either. They're the babies that are being

> adopted that were drug addicted, that don't necessarily have really severe, like, micro-preemie issues, so we don't have to worry about NEC [necrotizing enterocolitis].[2] So, the milk banks don't have enough milk so they don't prioritize them. But, one of the babies that I got to donate to had a cleft palate issue among some other really severe health issues. So, it wasn't severe enough that a milk bank would give breastmilk to them, and the parents couldn't necessarily pay the three bucks an ounce or whatever crazy amount it is to purchase breastmilk from the milk bank either. So, Get Pumped is kind of filling in a really important hole, so that's one of the reasons. Also, it's just less work for me. I don't need to do anything, I just pump and I drop off my milk and they get it to the right people. So, it's just easy and so I do that, but I also have people who have been coming to pick up my milk too, so I do both.'

When asked if she considered donating to Mothers' Milk Bank of Florida, Jane replied:

> 'I mean, I would if I had enough milk, but I'm really happy with my donation situation now. I think I'm filling a hole that a lot of people don't know about. Women know about milk banks. So, I mean, I do try to support them. I ran in the 5K to raise money for the milk bank and everything but what I'm doing I think is pretty much just as important as what Mothers' Milk Bank does. I'm just doing it in a different way.'

Jane's story highlights the reasons many donors give directly to recipients or through Get Pumped rather than through a milk bank, corroborating other research findings (Gribble 2013; Perrin et al 2016). Based on their belief in the superiority of breastmilk compared with infant formula, they wish to give their milk to babies whose needs are unmet by milk banks. Get Pumped makes it easy to ensure that donated milk is going to infants who need it, since the organization screens recipients and manages distribution of milk, but Jane also gives directly to other recipients whose needs are unmet by both other forms of milk distribution. In our online survey, which was conducted before the local milk bank opened, participants also indicated a preference for local donation rather than shipping their milk out of state (the nearest milk bank at the time was in North Carolina), a preference identified in other research (Gribble 2013; Perrin et al 2016). This preference for local sharing coupled with a desire to connect interpersonally through milk (Figure 3.1) and help babies who would not otherwise receive human milk are features that attract donors to milk sharing bio-communities of practice.

Gribble (2013) identified that many donors in her study held philosophical objections to milk banking, a theme that is also evident in our study. One critique participants held of milk banks, which emerged in the excerpt from Jane quoted earlier, is the financial cost. Several participants throughout our study critiqued the financial cost of banked milk, suggesting that it is prohibitive for some parents. Participants chose peer donation because they wanted to provide milk for babies whose parents were unable to afford it otherwise. However, this critique is somewhat misplaced, as hospitals and insurance companies most commonly bear the cost of banked milk (Perrin et al

Figure 3.1: Giving the gift of milk

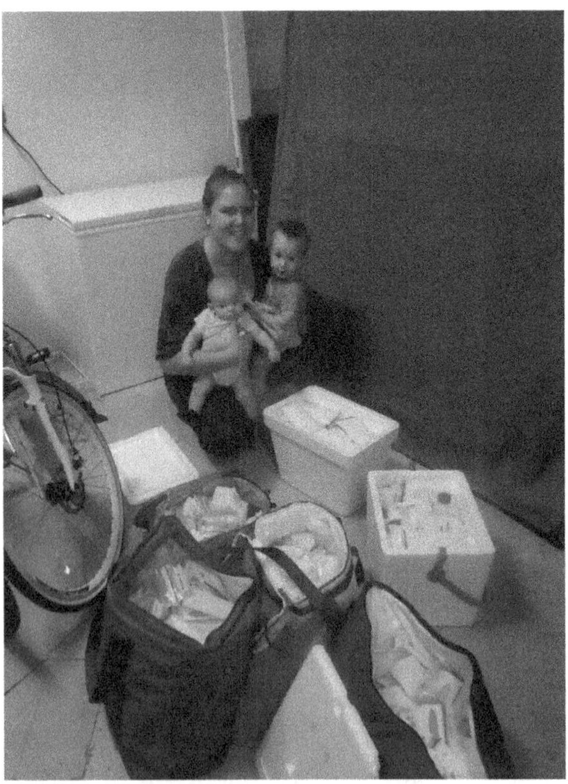

Source: Courtesy of Greta Nisbet

2016). Peer donors also critiqued the strict screening procedures used at milk banks. Jane continued:

> 'I've heard of things like moms will be taking a mild antidepressant that has been scientifically proven to not even show up in breastmilk at all and they won't be able to donate to a regular milk bank. But that doesn't mean that their milk is not good and it's not important and useful in other situations.'

Others critiqued the pasteurization process that takes place at milk banks. Louise, who served as a gestational surrogate twice and continued pumping milk to donate after both surrogate births, summarized as follows:

> 'I realized there were these whole communities of people that wanted the milk. I knew I didn't want to go through a milk bank because of the pasteurization process and then they're charging these moms. And it shouldn't be something that they have to pay so much money for.'

Various aspects of Jane's experience led to her becoming a central member of several milk sharing bio-communities of practice. The volume of her contribution, totalling in the thousands of ounces, meant that a comparatively large amount of her biological material was consumed by recipient babies. Her milk also had a relatively wide impact, being distributed to more than a dozen recipients. Through her professional activities as well as her donation practices, she was a well-known and recommended donor within several overlapping networks. She also embodied the situated knowledge and core values central to the milk sharing bio-communities she navigated. As a CLC, she was educated on the scientific properties of breastmilk and their beneficial impact on human infants. While she appreciated the important work of milk banks, she valued the distribution of unprocessed milk through Get Pumped and peer networks as complementary mechanisms for providing milk to babies who do not qualify for banked milk. Thus, she embodied the situated knowledge and core values necessary for the continuation of peer milk sharing.

About 40% of donors in our study who gave because they had abundant milk were occasional donors, giving milk only a few times when they happened to have excess. These mothers expressed milk with the intention of feeding it to their own children, ended up with more than they needed, and, on discovering peer milk sharing, they gave their excess to a peer recipient. Mothers in this category donated only to one or a few recipients, and they typically donated to each recipient only once. They described wanting their breastmilk to go to good use and not be wasted, but they did not work to continually express extra milk just to donate it.

Ashley experienced difficulties breastfeeding her second child, Chloe. As a newborn, Chloe had trouble latching on and was not efficient at extracting milk from Ashley's breast. Ashley began pumping to maintain the breastfeeding relationship and fed Chloe some of her expressed milk until she became better at nursing. Once Ashley and Chloe's breastfeeding relationship was established, Ashley had excess bags of expressed milk stored in her freezer. She described her first experience donating milk:

> 'I want to say maybe Chloe was two-and-a-half, three months the first time I shared milk. I had issues with Chloe in the beginning, nursing. I was pumping a lot of milk for her and eventually she got better at nursing, so I had milk in the freezer and the chiropractor that I take Chloe to, Leila, had a mom in need. So, I donated like 40 ounces 'cause I had so much stocked up from Chloe now nursing well and me getting ready to go back to work, I just had more than I even needed pumped. So that was my first experience.'

Like other donors with abundant milk who became occasional donors, Ashley ended up with excess bags of frozen milk that she expressed to feed to her own child but ended up not needing it. Hearing of a mother who needed milk for her baby, she decided to donate.

Ashley learned about peer milk sharing from a health professional, a common theme in our data. Among the 23 donors we interviewed, nearly half (48%, N=11) first learned about milk sharing from a healthcare professional, most commonly a midwife, chiropractor, doula, or lactation consultant. Another 48% (N=11) learned about milk sharing from peers, either through interactions on Facebook, face-to-face conversations with friends or family, or at support groups focused on mothering or breastfeeding. The remaining participant (4%, N=1) learned about milk sharing through a Google search to figure out something useful to do with her excess milk. The prevalence of healthcare providers facilitating peer breastmilk sharing is just starting to emerge in the research literature. Whereas some studies of peer milk sharing have reported little involvement of healthcare providers

(Perrin et al 2016; Falls 2017), one study aiming to assess the prevalence of peer milk use among mothers with low milk supply found that many who used peer milk received information about it from medical professionals, including pediatricians, midwives, nurses and lactation specialists (Cassar-Uhl and Liberatos 2018). In the communities we studied, the presence of the organization Get Pumped might have facilitated healthcare provider involvement, as several providers participated in the organization by referring donors and recipients, and allowed their offices to serve as breastmilk drop off, storage and pick-up sites. On the other hand, one interviewee – Madeline, a local midwife who collects breastmilk from donors she has screened and distributes it to recipients in her practice – recounted sharing milk within her circle of breastfeeding friends in 1996, when they would feed each other's babies as needed. Although Madeline allowed Get Pumped to use the freezers at her local birth centres as drop-off and pick-up locations, most of the milk that moved through her offices were coordinated by her, and not affiliated with the organization.

Ashley learned about peer milk sharing from Dr Leila, a chiropractor who is known by many in local natural parenting communities for her experience working with pregnant mothers, infants and children. She hosts monthly breastfeeding support groups at her office and is active in promoting breastfeeding, chiropractic care, exercise, nutrition and natural remedies. Dr Leila's office also serves as a drop-off, storage and pick-up site for Get Pumped. On learning about milk sharing from Dr Leila, who was collecting breastmilk to distribute to a local mother, Ashley donated the extra 40 ounces of milk she had in her freezer. She dropped the milk off to Dr Leila, who passed it on to the mother in need.

Later, Ashley donated more milk through Dr Leila for a different cause. She continued:

> 'Then there was, I think it might have been a month later, but there was a mom that had died in a car accident in another state. And the grandparents were asking for milk because the baby had only been breastfed and it wasn't taking formula at all. So, Dr Leila got as much milk as she could together to send to the family. So, I donated more milk then, whatever I had. I always usually keep about 20 ounces or so for Chloe. I don't need a lot because I pump it enough at work. And then there was another mom who wasn't able to nurse at all. She lives in Orlando and I gave her milk. Just once I shared with her. I think that was the last time that I shared milk.'

Although initiated into milk sharing through Dr Leila, Ashley later sought out recipients by posting online in a private Facebook group that she had excess milk to donate. She donated to each recipient just once, totalling about 120 ounces altogether. When asked if she had ever donated to the same baby multiple times, Ashley responded:

> 'No. It's all been different. The one mom that lives in Orlando – I just completely forgot her name because I'm horrible with names – I was going to donate again to her, but it was hard to get the milk to her because she lived in Orlando, which is about a half hour from here with traffic. So that didn't work out. So no, I don't think it's been multiple times, it's been different babies.'

Like other donors in this subcategory, Ashley donated when she had extra milk, but she did not develop long-term donating relationships with her recipients. She was casual in her approach to talking about milk sharing, as she forgot recipients' names, and only later in the interview remembered that she had a fourth recipient. At the time of our interview, she did not plan to donate any more milk because she was "not pumping any extra at all". Thus, when she happened to pump extra, she was happy to give it, but she did not pump specifically for giving. Nevertheless, she enjoyed being able to give to babies in need. When describing her donation experiences, she added:

> 'I mean, it feels great to be able to give milk. If I have it and it's there, why not share it with another baby in need? And I mean, I think with my son I probably would've been like, "No, I'd never take milk from somebody else." But now, I mean, just with sharing the milk and seeing the babies thrive and knowing they're getting the best, I would definitely, with Chloe, I would openly take milk if I needed to for her.... I joined some of the groups where moms share milk and just to see the whole community helping each other, it was definitely different than what I thought.'

Intending to give

In contrast to donors who produced excess milk and then decided to donate it, donors in the intending to give category decided they would become donors first, and then worked to produce extra milk for donation. They became routine donors who established pumping schedules that allowed them to give milk on a regular basis. Consistent with previous research on mothers who donate to milk banks (Arnold and Borman 1996; Azema and Callahan 2003; Osbaldiston and Mingle 2007; de Alencar and Seidle 2009; Carroll 2015; Oreg 2019) and those who share milk with peers (Shaw 2010, 2017, 2019; Gribble 2014b, 2018; Palmquist 2015; Perrin et al 2016; Falls 2017; Shaw and Morgan 2017; Wilson 2018), most participants in this category described their desire to give breastmilk as a way of helping others. In contrast to portrayals of breastmilk donors in popular press and some academic literature as women who just automatically – with no planning, preparation, or additional labour – have extra milk to give (Carter et al 2015), we find that some wish to become breastmilk donors before ever producing excess milk.

Raven was unaware of peer milk sharing when she breastfed her first two children, but she experienced oversupply with both. She had some familiarity with milk banks, but the work involved in packaging and shipping milk to North Carolina where it would be processed and distributed did not appeal to her. While pregnant with her third child, she learned about Get Pumped and decided then to become a donor. She explained:

> 'With my first two babies I didn't know there was really an option to donate. It wasn't close, a local option, it was national milk banks. Whereas with this pregnancy my really good friend was an International Board Certified Lactation Consultant. And she had posted it on her Facebook and I was like, "Oh what is that?" And then I read about the organization Get Pumped. And so, then I messaged her and said, "Can I become a donor before I even have the baby? Can I sign up now?" And she said, "Sure, go ahead." And I was like, "Well, at least my milk is going somewhere."'

When asked why she became a donor, Raven continued:

> 'Because I have an oversupply of milk. And I can't lower my milk supply. Like, most women could just not pump and ignore it and their milk supply lessens, but if I don't pump my body just goes, "Oh, let's make some more milk until she can't ignore us anymore." And so, I have to pump to be comfortable. So, I just started pumping and donating. With my boys I actually had to take medication to stop making so much milk.'

Anticipating that she would have excess milk based on her past experience, Raven decided to become a breastmilk donor, completing the application process for Get Pumped, and becoming a member of milk sharing bio-communities of practice before she even had milk to give. At the time of our interview, she had been donating about 100 ounces of milk each month.

Raven explained that she takes pride in her status as a milk donor. She documented her journey by photographing her bags of frozen milk before each donation, and posting them on Facebook, a common practice for donors and recipients alike. She explained:

> 'I post pictures of my big milk bag when I fill it up, with the number of ounces. And it's not really to brag about it, it's more like my personal journey of donating milk. And I want to keep track and so it's my way of tracking it. I can go back and look at all my pictures and go, "Okay, I donated this many ounces altogether."'

Donating milk provided a sense of personal satisfaction for Raven. None of her friends donated milk, so she did not consider herself part of a milk-sharing community. Likewise, she did not connect her donation to any form of spirituality or sense of religious purpose. She received positive reinforcement for her donations from significant others, but for her milk sharing is more of an individual journey, focused on her personal identity rather than her integration in a social network. Because she donates only to Get Pumped, she does not establish intimate relationships with her recipients. Instead, her connection is more abstract, similar to the 'imagined communities' of donors and recipients of banked milk that Tanya Cassidy and Abdullahi El Tom (2010) describe and that Rhonda Shaw notes in her research (Shaw and Morgan 2017; Shaw 2019). Nevertheless, Raven and other similar donors are significant members for the participants who receive their milk, as they contribute to their recipient babies' sustenance through their material donations, as well as to the continuation of the bio-communities of practice to which they donate. Their milk is imbued with emotive value, as it is symbolic of their moral identities and their intentions to help babies in need.

Another pathway to becoming a milk donor within the intending to give category, which was less common yet still prevalent, is a desire to 'give back'. These participants had been breastmilk recipients at some previous time, and although they were not giving directly to those from whom they had received, they became breastmilk donors as a way of giving back. They viewed their breastmilk donations as a form of reciprocity, a way of giving back to the community that had generously provided for them.

Christine had taken in a foster baby, Liam, for whom she received breastmilk from about 40 donors, enabling her to feed him breastmilk until he was two years old. I (Shannon) had met Christine and Liam briefly at a Baby Expo in Orlando and learned a little bit about their story. A couple months later, Christine was close to running out of milk, and Dr Leila, our mutual friend and chiropractor, recommended me as a potential donor. Christine contacted me through Facebook messenger, asking if I had any milk to give. I gathered up all of the milk I had, which was about 85 ounces, and we set up a time for Christine to come to my house that afternoon to pick it up. We met in my garage, were my secondary freezer is, chatted for a few minutes, and I gave her the milk. We continued to participate in the same online communities, so I knew that Christine had become pregnant and given birth to another baby. During a subsequent research meeting, when Beatriz described her most recent interview, I knew immediately it was Christine. "I know exactly who you're talking about!," I exclaimed. "I donated to her!" That special connection I felt to this participant despite meeting in person only twice illustrates the emotional materiality of milk, particularly its ability to bond communities of people together.

Now that she had given birth to her own biological child and was able to produce breastmilk, Christine became a peer milk donor as a way of giving back. She decided that she would give her milk long before she gave birth to her baby. She sought out adopted babies to give to because she felt particularly sympathetic toward adoptive parents and wanted to help these babies receive breastmilk. When Beatriz asked what led her to start giving milk, Christine explained:

> 'Because I was given so much milk, I wanted to do it. I told my husband one of my goals is to be able to give a thousand ounces to an adopted baby, over the course – I want to have a few more children – so over the course of all my pregnancies and births, I want to be able to say that I gave a thousand ounces to specifically an adopted baby. Because that's what was given to me. And I feel like when you adopt a baby, you really don't have any other options. It's not like you're just working and you have to pump or

> something like that, you really have no other option. So, I feel like they are some of the most desperate of everybody in the community that's looking for milk. And so, I have just been pumping a little bit every day since my daughter was born two months ago, just saving it because – I didn't know why. And that's when a friend called me up and said, "Oh my gosh, I just adopted a baby. She's screaming! She's crazy! Blah, blah, blah." And I said, "Well, have you thought about breastmilk?" And she's like, "Well it's funny you should mention it. Only today, somebody else mentioned it to me." And so I said, "Well, I've got, you know, enough for a day or two if you want to try it." And so that's how that got started.'

Christine's explanation of why she became a breastmilk donor highlights her desire to reciprocate what was given to her. Over the course of feeding her foster baby donated milk, she estimated that she was given around a thousand ounces, and she wished to give back the same amount.

Christine's prolonged immersion and extensive connectedness contribute to her position as a central member of the milk-sharing bio-communities of practice in which she participated. At the time of her interview, she had already been involved in the communities for a few years, establishing bio-intimate connections with the vast number of donors who gave their milk to her as well as those who were now receiving her milk. She adhered to the central norms of the groups, following established screening and milk-handling guidelines, and rejected the commodification of human milk. Christine also deliberately gave her milk to peers rather than donating to Get Pumped or Mothers' Milk Bank of Florida because she valued the relationships she built through milk sharing. She explained, "I wanted to have a relationship. If I was going to donate to somebody, I wanted to have more of a relationship with them instead of just donating it to a regular milk bank or something. I wanted to know them and see why they needed it and stuff like that." She explained that these personal relationships provided incentive to continue pumping because, "I knew that my breastmilk was going to a child who actually really needed it." Thus, the personal connections established through milk-sharing bio-communities of practice can incentivize donors to continue their participation (Gribble 2013, 2014b; Falls 2017).

Giving by request

The final path to becoming a peer milk donor among our study participants was giving by request. This is the pathway that led me (Shannon) to become a peer milk donor. When I was breastfeeding Ella, my second child, a friend from the breastfeeding support group I attended at the birth centre where Ella was born was collecting milk for a mother whose baby was diagnosed as failing to thrive. Hailey called me one day after a group meeting that I had missed, and described Jackson, a frail baby who was brought to the group by his mother, Sheila, who was experiencing difficulties breastfeeding. Hailey had breastfed the baby to see if he was able to extract milk. He was, so they assumed Sheila was not producing. Hailey was collecting as much breastmilk as she could for Sheila – who did not want to feed her baby formula – and asked if I had any to spare. Ella was about six months old by then, and my milk had levelled out to where I was producing enough for her and pumping while I was at work, but I had to work to keep enough milk for her in the freezer, and my partner used extreme care not to waste any. I did not consider myself someone who had excess milk, but I also felt compelled to help baby Jackson, and I felt sorry for Sheila. While Hailey and I were still on the phone, I assessed my breastmilk stash, which consisted of about two four-ounce bottles in the refrigerator and ten four-ounce bags of frozen milk in the freezer. I quickly reasoned that if Ella could drink the refrigerated milk while I was at work the next day, and I could use the weekend to start replenishing the freezer milk for use the following week, I could give all of the milk that was in my freezer to Jackson. I delivered the milk to Hailey that day, who passed it on, along with the other milk she collected.

Similar to others in this category, I became a breastmilk donor when someone requested my milk. Although I had already been introduced to milk sharing when I was asked to participate, some mothers in this category were unaware of the practice until it was requested of them. Some happened across a post requesting milk on Facebook, either by a friend or in a private group, whereas others were asked directly by a close friend or family member. Most, like me, did not necessarily view themselves as someone who had excess milk to share, but when asked, decided that they could spare some of their milk. For some, this entry into peer milk sharing led to them becoming routine donors, whereas others became only occasional donors, giving when an apparent need emerged yet not seeking out long-term donation relationships.

Allison became a peer milk donor in response to a request for breastmilk she saw on Facebook. At the time of the interview, Allison had donated to five recipients, which included four babies and a male friend of a friend who used her milk to treat his psoriasis. She told us the story of how she first learned about milk sharing and became a donor:

> 'Someone had posted in a group that I'm in on Facebook that they needed some milk for their baby. And I have a really good supply, so I had a lot in my freezer. So, I'm like, well, I think I can spare some. So, I gave her some. And I don't have a whole lot of room in my freezer so I make sure I have at least 100 ounces in my freezer and usually once I hit 200 I'm like, okay, I have to get rid of some of this. So sometimes I'll message anybody that I've shared with and I'll be like, "Do you need any?"'

Characteristic of mothers in this category, and in contrast to mainstream portrayals of milk-sharing participants, Allison did not seek breastmilk sharing as a way of managing excess milk. Instead, she became a peer milk donor when prompted by someone who was looking for milk. She then became an occasional donor, giving milk whenever she had extra milk to give. At the time of our interview, she had given around 400 ounces, and planned to continue donating as long as she had extra. When asked how she typically finds recipients, Allison continued:

> 'I guess all of them have pretty much been through Facebook, really. Because I'm in a local moms' group. It's usually people from that group. And then the other was just a friend from work who knows that I breastfeed and so she just asked me if I ever donated my milk for anything, so I donated to her.'

Although Allison has not become friends with her recipients, they were initially connected through their mutual membership in a virtual community. She explained that, from a larger 'private' group with around 600 members, a smaller 'secret' group emerged with around 200 members. On Facebook, a private group can be found by anyone who searches for it, but individuals must request to become members. A secret group is one that cannot be identified by non-members, and therefore members can only be added by other members. It is through this secret group that Allison identified and established relationships with her recipients. Although Allison gave milk only on occasion, she embraced the core ideologies of the bio-communities, giving her milk away for free, and never turning away a potential recipient, because, as she explained, "I can't really think of anything that would make me say, 'No, I can't give your baby my milk.'" She posted milk-sharing memes and information about her own involvement openly on Facebook, educating others in her broader social network about the practice. She became known for her role as a peer milk donor and 'lactivist', as she was regularly tagged by others on articles or posts related to breastfeeding and milk sharing.

Similarly, Louise also became a breastmilk donor by request. She explained:

> 'I think the first time I donated milk was when my daughter was about a year-and-a-half old. I had a friend that was adopting from overseas and wanted to induce lactation. And basically, I wanted to help her segue into that instead of having a baby that was artificially fed while she was working on the breastfeeding and everything, at least to have breastmilk be familiar.'

Later on, Louise became a surrogate and, after giving birth, expressed milk solely for donation. She continued:

> 'Then when I actually met Thelma [one of Louise's later breastmilk recipients who participated in a co-interview with Beatriz] and I was actually a surrogate a few years ago and afterwards the parents wanted the milk for a couple of weeks and then that was it. And I was pumping, pumping, and pumping. I was like, "I need to empty out my freezer." So that's how Thelma and I met initially. And there were a couple other moms then I was donating to, for about a three-month period, until I weaned off the pumping. And then I did another surrogacy recently, so I was able to donate to Thelma again for another child. And it was kind of the same process of reaching out, saying, "This is what I have, this is what's available, this is my medical history."'

Although Louise initially became a peer milk donor by the request of her friend, over time she became a central participant, donating to at least a dozen recipients, and establishing long-term relationships with many of them. Like Beatriz' donor, Jill, she pumped for several months after giving birth to her two surrogate babies, solely for the purpose of donating milk. Although Louise initially became a milk donor based on peer request, she later donated again based on her desire to give babies breastmilk, becoming more like participants in the intending to give category, demonstrating that individuals' motivations and circumstances can change over time. As many women give birth to more than one child, their roles in peer milk-sharing bio-communities can shift, a phenomenon also noted by Falls (2017).

Becoming a recipient

For caretakers who engage in the receiving end of milk sharing, entrance into the bio-communities of practice occurs in several ways, though all begin with an infant who, for whatever reason, is unable to consume their mother's own milk. In the US, peer breastmilk recipients most commonly obtain expressed frozen milk from donors, which they thaw, heat and then feed to their babies through a bottle or supplemental nursing system (SNS)[3] (Reyes-Foster et al 2015; Palmquist and Doehler 2016; Falls 2017; Wilson 2018) (Figures 3.2 and 3.3). Among our survey participants, about 22% of recipients also allowed their babies to be co-fed, directly breastfed by a peer donor. None of our participants *only* engaged in breastmilk sharing as a recipient of co-feeding but used this form of milk sharing in conjunction with others, either by also receiving expressed frozen milk, co-feeding someone else's baby, or donating frozen milk. By contrast, nearly half of participants who reported ever being a recipient of peer breastmilk *only* engaged in peer milk sharing by receiving expressed frozen milk.

Parents and other caregivers become breastmilk recipients through a variety of paths, yet they share a commitment to feeding their children breastmilk and an inability to provide it on their own (Thorley 2012; Gribble 2014c; Palmquist and Doehler 2014, 2016; Palmquist 2015; Reyes-Foster et al 2015; Falls 2017; Giles 2017; Cassar-Uhl and Liberatos 2018; Wilson 2018). While we did not encounter recipients who came into milk sharing through situations such as critical illness or death of the mother, some of our donors, such as Ashley, reported that they had gifted breastmilk in such situations, when the baby's father, grandparents or friends of the mother collected breastmilk based on the mother's wishes. Some, including Shannon, also gave to same-sex couples in circumstances of adoption, surrogacy, or where breastfeeding was undesired by the gestational parent. Other scholars have documented instances where transgender fathers give birth but

Figure 3.2: SNS in use

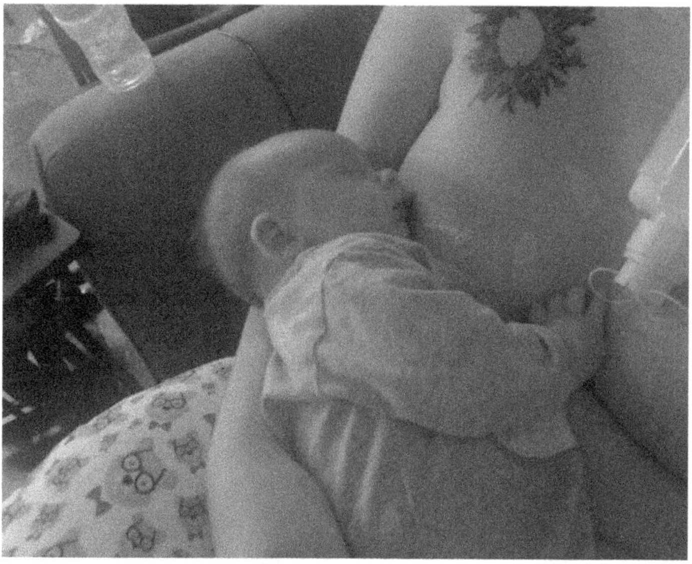

Source: Courtesy of Alex Ryan

experience difficulties chestfeeding as a result of chest surgery, and opt to receive peer milk (MacDonald et al 2016; Giles 2017; Wilson 2018). Among our study participants, the primary recipient parents were white, cisgender, heterosexual women who were committed to breastfeeding, but encountered breastfeeding difficulties. This was the case for 80% of recipients who participated in our in-depth interviews. The remaining 20% became parents through fostering or adoption. Like donors, participants also varied and shifted in being central or peripheral to the bio-communities of practice based not only on the amount of breastmilk or ability to exclusively feed an infant breastmilk, but also the degree of involvement in the process of obtaining milk and the establishment of relationships with other members. Just as donors initially came to milk sharing through abundant milk, intention and request, recipients similarly came to milk sharing through insufficient milk, intention and offers of milk. We explore these experiences in the following sections.

Insufficient milk

Consistent with previous research, the most common reason we encountered for seeking donated milk mirrored my (Beatriz') experience: insufficient milk supply. Rhonda shared her milk-sharing

Figure 3.3: Feeding baby donor milk

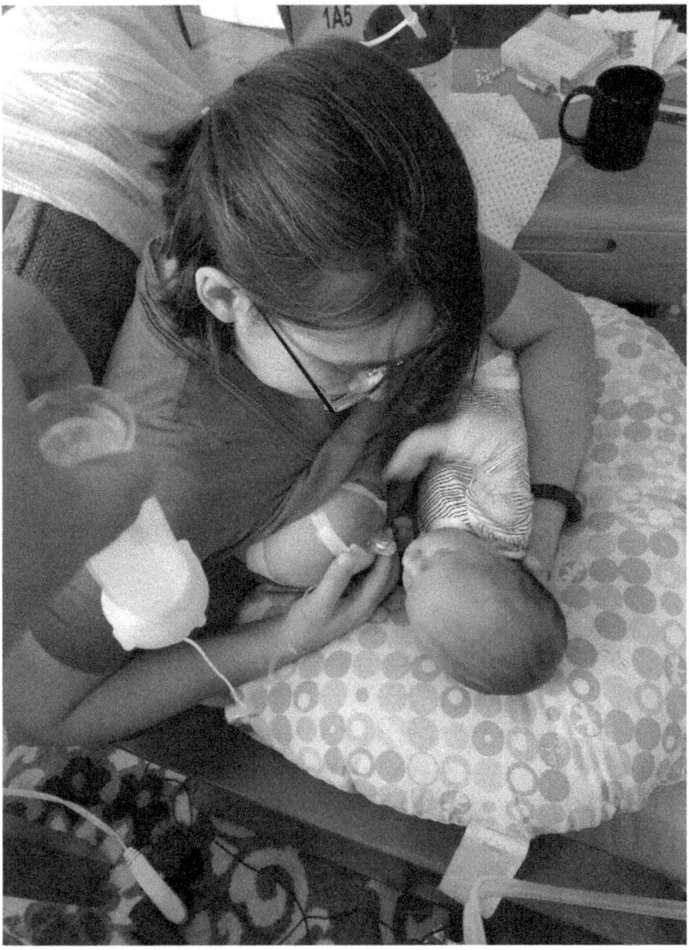

Source: Courtesy of E. A. Quinn

journey with me over iced tea shortly after giving birth to her third baby:

> 'With Marie [her first child], I had a C-section. It was traumatic. And so, anyway, I ended up having to use formula, and I just felt like a failure. I wasn't able to breastfeed her at all. I think my body was so in shock from the C-section I wasn't expecting. So anyway, I used formula, and I just didn't even, I didn't think much about it. And then, I thought about it, I was like, you know I tried to

> breastfeed as much as I could.... But I had a feeling, when I got pregnant with Susan, I felt like if I had just had a regular birth, or a home birth, I should be able to breastfeed. Like, it was gonna happen. I thought, "Oh, it'll happen for sure!" And so, I did, I had a home birth with Susan, and then I had the same exact issues that I had with Marie. So, I knew it wasn't the C-section's fault.'

Similar to my story, although Rhonda experienced difficulties breastfeeding her first child, she thought her experience the second time around would be much easier, especially if she was able to avoid a traumatic birth, which she blamed for her breastfeeding difficulties. Rhonda did give birth to her second child vaginally at home, so she was surprised when she encountered barriers to breastfeeding again. She explained that her breastfeeding difficulties led her to experience depression, "Because I thought for sure I'd be able to nurse just fine, and I wasn't." Many recipients in our study described breastfeeding challenges as wrought with emotion, swaying between frustration and anger to sadness and despair. They described being disappointed in their bodies for not producing enough milk and questioning themselves as mothers, common themes throughout breastfeeding research (Kelleher 2006; Lee 2007, 2008; Ryan et al 2010; Taylor and Wallace 2012; Schafer et al 2018). Many participants cried at this point during the interviews, and often, we cried with them.

Recipients described initially being in disbelief that their bodies were not producing enough milk. Like other participants, Rhonda described identifying a breastfeeding problem as an unfolding process. She explained:

> 'At first people thought, "Oh, it's Susan, she has a lip-tie, probably." Or, you know, "Her mouth isn't strong enough."'Cause she was born three weeks early, but that's still full-term. So, I took her to her paediatrician and had her mouth tested, and they said, "Yes, her mouth is weak." But I still didn't think so because I felt like her latch was really good.... But she wasn't gaining weight so I had to do the weight checks. I was very stressed out. She had, she was jaundiced, and so the doctors were pressuring me to give her formula, because they said formula takes the jaundice out because it does something to the system, which, you know, it was very hard for me to believe them. I just didn't believe that. But anyway, I would put her on the breast for

> 40 minutes, 50 minutes, an hour, and she would just be suckling, falling asleep, but she wasn't gaining any weight. And, then there was a time, maybe when she was a little bit older, where she would just go on the breast, and she would just be screaming. I actually breastfed her for maybe four months, which is a long time compared to Marie, which was just a couple weeks that I tried. So, I was getting a little bit of milk but it wasn't enough to sustain her, as far as I could tell.... And I was pumping too after every feeding, I was doing everything. I even took Domperidone and I took Susan to the chiropractor, I went to the chiropractor, I did acupuncture. I had an IBCLC come out and spend a whole day with me and watch what I was doing. And I was doing everything – she was like, "You're doing everything right," she's like, "You're doing a really good job."'

Rhonda's story highlights the process involved over the span of a few months through which she figured out that her baby was not getting enough milk. Like other mothers who are strongly committed to breastfeeding, Rhonda approached breastfeeding as a 'carefully managed project' (Avishai 2007) and sought professional, medical and alternative assistance (Andrews and Knaak 2013; Torres 2014). She believed in her own ability to breastfeed her child. When things did not go as planned, she consulted multiple health providers to assess her baby, observe her breastfeeding techniques, and, through chiropractic care and acupuncture, correct any malalignment that could interfere with breastfeeding. She tried many different techniques to increase her milk supply, including taking the prescription medication Domperidone, which is understood to increase breastmilk production, but is not USFDA-approved. She pumped after every feeding to increase the demand on her body to produce milk. Like other recipients, Rhonda was extremely committed to breastfeeding her baby, and worked very hard to achieve her goals. Despite her efforts, she was unable to meet her baby's needs.

Rhonda explained that she learned about peer milk sharing after she had already switched her first baby, Marie, to formula. Feeling traumatized by Marie's cesarean birth, Rhonda sought support from the local chapter of ICAN, which holds meetings at a local coffee shop one evening each month. During her attendance at the meetings, she observed some of the other participants engaging in peer milk sharing, as some milk-sharing participants would meet at the ICAN meetings and transfer milk there. Rhonda thought this was a great idea, and held in the back of her mind that if she had difficulties breastfeeding future babies she would prefer to use peer breastmilk instead of formula. However, she believed this would be unnecessary, especially if she was able to avoid a cesarean in any subsequent births. After about four months of breastfeeding Susan but feeling that she was not getting enough milk, Rhonda decided to ask a friend to breastfeed Susan as a way of assessing the baby's ability to extract milk from a breast.

> 'So, I had taken her to the paediatrician who thought her mouth was weak, and then I asked one of my friends if she could nurse Susan and see if she felt like Susan was pulling milk out. And so, she did, and Susan was just fine. Her latch was good, and I felt that way too. I feel like, when you're a mother, you know something's going on. And so, I felt like Susan was fine nursing, and she was, she was able to take milk from my friend, and was totally content and happy. She wasn't screaming, because there was enough milk there, because my friend was nursing, you know? And so, I was like, "Okay, so she's not pulling off and screaming with her." And so, I just kind of felt like I wasn't making enough milk.'

The fact that Susan was able to successfully breastfeed from Rhonda's friend and appear content and happy as a result confirmed Rhonda's suspicion that she was not producing enough milk. Rhonda began seeking milk from peers to meet Susan's nutritional needs while avoiding the use of formula. Altogether, she received milk from seven donors to feed Susan. Some became long-term donors, providing milk on a regular basis for several months, whereas others gave milk only once or twice. Rhonda's third baby, Jaime, was born prematurely and spent several weeks in the NICU. He received banked human milk, and Rhonda pumped her own milk to feed him as well. Once he reached a certain weight, he was no longer eligible for banked milk, at which point the hospital personnel supplemented Rhonda's milk with formula. Rhonda received offers of breastmilk for Jaime, which she accepted and brought into the hospital and continued to feed to him at home. However, since Rhonda believed that Jaime was doing well on formula, and she was busier now that she had three children, she did less to actively seek peer milk. At the time that Beatriz sat down with Rhonda for an interview, Jaime was five months old and was drinking one bottle of donated milk each day and the rest formula. He had received milk from five donors.

Rhonda's milk-sharing journey demonstrates the way in which members' degrees of participation and involvement in milk sharing bio-communities of practice is an unfolding and changing process. When she first became aware of milk sharing, Rhonda was a peripheral member of the bio-communities – she knew one site where milk sharing took place and resolved that, if needed, she would one day seek out donor milk. Once she realized that she was not producing enough milk for Susan, Rhonda became a central member of the bio-communities, actively seeking milk from several sources in order to exclusively feed her baby shared milk. Once Jaime was born, she became a peripheral participant once again, feeding her baby breastmilk as much as she could but not to the degree that she did with Susan.

Mothers who experienced insufficient milk or other breastfeeding difficulties did not originally set out to use shared milk. Their original intention had been to exclusively breastfeed their own babies, but when supplementation became necessary they somehow became aware that they had another option besides formula. Healthcare and other types of birth-care providers were key to making new mothers aware of milk sharing as an option – although I (Beatriz) was already aware of milk sharing because of my research, this option was brought up with me by my doula and my midwife when I started having difficulty with supply. Other interview respondents – Anna, Mona Lisa, and Shirley – reported learning about milk sharing from a doula or lactation consultant. Social media – most notably Facebook groups – also played an important role in exposing recipients to milk sharing. Samantha and Jackie both learned about milk sharing this way.

The perceived vitality of breastmilk informs the ways milk-sharing participants talk about human milk versus artificial formula. Several of our participants who received gifted milk also used formula at some point, either before they discovered peer milk sharing, or when they were unable to acquire enough breastmilk from peers to fully avoid it. Recipients who did feed their babies formula tended to report negative effects they observed in their babies that they attributed to formula, such as digestive problems or 'gassiness'. They also reported substantial differences in the form, texture and smell of their babies' faeces when they consumed formula compared to breastmilk, which they interpreted as further evidence of the superiority of breastmilk. Mona Lisa explained, "It's only been a couple days that I'd have to give him formula and I could tell, he starts getting gassy. He doesn't get as bad as the first time but, you know, very gassy, and his poop, he starts getting very constipated." Falls (2017) refers to these observed differences as the 'poo oracle' that served as evidence for herself as a peer breastmilk recipient and for the parents she spoke with of the superiority of peer breastmilk over infant formula. New mothers are often told they should look for 'grainy, mustard-like poo' in their babies' diapers. The pasty, fetid faeces produced by formula-fed infants was a source of distress and disappointment for mothers who were committed to breastfeeding and had to resort to formula.

Based on these beliefs about the benefits of breastmilk over formula, breastmilk recipients reported an unwavering commitment to breastfeeding their babies, describing breastfeeding as a "passion", and some identifying as "breastfeeding advocates" or "lactivists". However, these mothers' breastfeeding journeys did not go as planned. Many, like Anna, whose story we present in Chapter 2, faced a combination of health and societal obstacles that made exclusive breastfeeding impossible. They experienced a variety of breastfeeding difficulties, ranging from issues with the baby having tongue-tie, lip-tie[4] or a weak suck that interfered with their ability to extract milk from the breast, to insufficient milk production for reasons that were unknown or attributed to some other health condition such as thyroid dysfunction or polycystic ovary syndrome. Several recipients, like Rhonda and Beatriz, who had multiple children experienced breastfeeding difficulties with their previous child(ren), yet initially believed they would have greater success with a subsequent child.

Rhonda's story closely resembles that of Beatriz. Like Beatriz, Rhonda was convinced her body could and would produce enough milk to sustain her babies, and that the initial difficulties were due to her traumatic birth experience. Both Beatriz and Rhonda, like many of our participants, experienced deep feelings of sadness and failure when they realized they could not produce enough milk for their infants. Their surprise at being unable to breastfeed turned into feelings of betrayal by their own bodies and failure. Both became central participants in their bio-communities of practice by engaging in extensive investment of time, money and labour to obtain peer milk for their babies. Likewise, as their lives became more complicated, they also recognized the significant investment of time and other resources involved in feeding a baby exclusively with donor milk, and were comfortable with feeding their third babies formula, thus becoming peripheral members. Throughout their narratives, recipient mothers explained that they had "done everything right" and made every effort, including significant financial sacrifice, to exclusively breastfeed their own babies. It was only after all other options had been exhausted that donor milk became an option they would consider. The journey was painful and full of sadness and regret alongside relief – milk sharing thus allows women with breastfeeding difficulties to alleviate feelings of shame and regret associated with being unable to breastfeed (McCloskey and Karandikar 2019; Schafer et al 2018). The emotional language used to describe donor breastmilk, alongside feelings of joy at seeing the physiological changes in their baby's body (and excretions) as a result, points to the emotional materiality of breastmilk at the heart of these bio-communities of practice.

Intending to receive

Although the majority of our research participants were biological mothers who attempted, unsuccessfully, to exclusively breastfeed their babies, two of our interview participants and several in our online survey were adoptive mothers who intended to feed their babies peer-shared milk from the very beginning. While they did not undergo the physical experience of pregnancy and subsequent lactation, they still desired to feed their adoptive or foster babies breastmilk. Of these two recipients, one of them, Christine, whose story is explored earlier in this chapter, took on both roles of donor and recipient at different points in time in her parenting journey.

Olivia's son Emerson was seven years old when baby Adelyn came to live with them at only eight days old. Olivia had breastfed Emerson until he self-weaned at 21 months, so she was already strongly committed to breastfeeding. A single mother, she tried hard to have a second baby, undergoing several rounds of fertility treatments and experiencing three miscarriages. Just as she was preparing to do another round of fertility treatment, she received word that she had been selected by an adoption agency to have Adelyn placed with her. She cancelled her fertility appointment and took in Adelyn instead. After only six days, Adelyn's biological parents wanted her back, so Olivia had to give her up. Nine days later Adelyn came back to live with Olivia and Emerson for good. Several months later, Olivia was able to formally adopt Adelyn.

Being committed to breastfeeding, Olivia took Domperidone to induce lactation, and supplemented her own milk with formula that she fed to Adelyn through an SNS, which allows the baby to latch onto the mother's breast to stimulate milk production, yet receive both whatever breastmilk is produced along with some formula that comes through a tube attached to the mother's nipple (Figures 3.2 and 3.3). This system teaches babies to latch on to the breast, while rewarding them with milk even if the mother's body is not producing enough. It also facilitates the physical closeness and skin-to-skin contact understood to promote emotional bonding and stimulate milk production. Olivia fed Adelyn this way for several weeks, pumping whatever milk she could during her lunch breaks and her commute back and forth to work. Despite her efforts, she was not able to produce much of her own milk. Olivia was first introduced to peer milk sharing at an infant massage class she took when Adelyn was about three months old. She met a mother in the class who had a little bit of extra colostrum in her freezer that she offered to donate. The donor introduced Olivia to a secret Facebook group geared toward natural parenting – the same group that Allison described – where Olivia found several other mothers who gave her milk. She learned more about milk sharing through this group and through her own internet research, and located several other donors through the state-level Facebook pages of Eats on Feets and Human Milk 4 Human Babies. By the time Olivia met with me (Shannon) at a café during her lunch break to talk about milk sharing, Adelyn was 14 months old, and had received milk from nine donors. Some donors gave only enough milk for a bottle or two, whereas others established long-term relationships, giving regularly for a span of several months. In this way, Olivia entered the bio-communities of practice and soon became a central member.

Having a child who was adopted, Olivia knew that she was given priority by some donors over other potential recipients. In recounting a few donors who were part of the Facebook group where she initially received milk, Olivia said, "It was great because I think all the moms, everyone knew I adopted so it was kind of like I became the first priority in this group of moms. Because they knew that I didn't have the milk whereas another mom, her supply is dropping but she has milk versus I didn't have any." Susan Falls also observed that adoptive parents are at the top of the 'hierarchy of need that structures the distribution of milk' (2017: 83), often given preference over others who seek milk. Adoptive parents in particular are viewed as 'worthy recipients' (Reyes-Foster and Carter 2018b) since they would not normally be expected to produce breastmilk on their own.

Receiving by offer

Just as some participants became donors when they encountered someone who needed milk, others became recipients when they were offered milk. This method of becoming a recipient was the least common in our study, occurring among just a handful of recipients who took our online survey. Some who obtained expressed milk were mothers who were breastfeeding, but struggled in some way, either from acute illness or difficulty pumping. On having their struggles recognized by a peer, they were offered breastmilk, which they accepted and fed to their babies. Caroline explained, "Several bouts of mastitis and an antibiotic reaction hurt my supply and I had to supplement. Several friends offered their milk to me, so I used it until I recovered." Where Caroline suffered from acute illness, Dena experienced short-term difficulties producing enough milk: "When my daughter was born premature, they wouldn't allow me a lot of skin-to-skin time in the hospital. Because of this my milk was difficult to pump. My friend brought me some of her milk so I wouldn't be forced into using formula." Whereas Caroline and Dena were offered milk to manage shorter-term obstacles, others were offered small amounts of milk to offset low milk supply. Francesca explained, "A friend had an overage of pumped milk she was afraid would go bad before she used it. She knew I had a hard time with milk supply and offered any milk her own son didn't use while she was at work." Helena had a similar experience: "I was taking a class and a friend saw I was pumping. She needed to pump as well and offered me her milk for my baby, as I didn't have much reserve supply. I was very thankful." Those who became recipients through offers of milk tended to receive only small amounts of milk for a short time frame.

A few participants who took our online survey became recipients through offers of direct co-feeding. These participants also acquired small amounts of milk only once or infrequently. For some, the offers were from friends, which allowed them to rest, work, or engage in occasional leisure activities, like attending a concert. Leslie stated, "My friend came and took my baby for the day so I could rest." Similarly, Sylvia explained, "My friend and I set up a date night swap. Both of our youngest children nursed so we would nurse when the other was out." One respondent, Monica, became a recipient in response to an emergency situation: "While on a trip to my aunt's house with a friend and her baby my aunt fell down the stairs. I didn't want to take my daughter to the germy hospital so my friend kept her and nursed her."

The stories presented in this chapter illustrate the many pathways to milk sharing that lead parents and caretakers to become members of milk sharing bio-communities of practice. These pathways lead potential donors and recipients to the bio-communities of practice locally available through both in-person encounters –such as hearing about milk sharing from a friend at an infant massage class or witnessing a milk exchange in a cesarean support meeting – and in virtual spaces such as private and secret Facebook groups or even more publicly visible Eats on Feets and Human Milk for Human Babies pages. These bio-communities of practice may overlap in membership and location, but their emergence tends to be organic, often the result of people sharing their experiences of struggle and others coming to their aid. As people become better acquainted with the etiquette and processes of breastmilk sharing, they become central to the bio-communities of practice. These processes of socialization and the practices involved are more fully explored in Chapter 4.

4

Milk-Sharing Practices

5.30 am. A baby stirs, then cries. His mother, Cassie, lying in bed beside him, latches him to her breast, half asleep, and the nursling settles. A few minutes later, she gets up and heads to her rocking chair in the room next door, where her double electric pump is set up. She sits down and starts her morning pumping routine, washing her hands beforehand and ensuring all of her pump parts are clean and sanitized. Twenty minutes later, after making sure she washes her hands again, she carefully transfers the milk to storage bags, lays them flat on a cookie sheet, and places them in the freezer. Once they freeze flat, she will stack them neatly and slide them into a gallon-sized storage bag that will go into a specially designated freezer in her garage. Throughout her day, she repeats this same routine at least four times. By the end of the week, her freezer will be full of gallon-sized zipper bags full of eight-ounce milk-storage bags. Some of the milk is meant for Get Pumped, but on any given week she might offer some up to a desperate mother posting on Human Milk 4 Human Babies, or to a friend of a friend who is just not making enough milk. Cassie is very proud of the fact that she produces thick, creamy milk – she calls it buttermilk – and she's sure the babies she has fed have benefitted greatly from it. Meeting babies who drink her milk, she says, "lights her heart on fire".

Meanwhile, in another part of town, another mother, Thelma, is also starting her day. Her own baby stirs, and she gets up to retrieve the bag of milk she left to defrost in her fridge the day before. She washes her hands, sighs in relief to see the bag didn't leak into the bowl it was sitting in, pours its contents into a bottle, and sets it into a bowl of warm water to heat it. She opens her freezer, frowns at the dwindling supply of frozen milk bags, and grabs her cell phone as she picks up the warmed bottle of donor milk and walks back to her bedroom to feed her baby. She logs on to a local Facebook group and posts some information about herself, her baby, and her need for milk.

She might choose one of her more recent pictures of her smiling baby to get potential donors' attention. If things go well, she may spend the rest of her day driving to meet donors. If they don't, she will post across different groups until she receives enough offers and she can rebuild her 'stash'. Once she gets a response, Thelma will send a friend request to potential donors and review three years of their online life before she accepts their offer. She will drive whatever distance she has to for milk, but she will only take milk from someone if she can meet their baby in person. When she meets a potential donor, she will quiz them on their milk-handling techniques. Every once in a while, something won't feel right. When this happens, she will thank the potential donor for their willingness to share and politely decline the milk. One time, she said, a donor insisted so much that she take her milk that she reluctantly accepted the milk and then threw it away. For her, there is nothing more important than ensuring what she puts into her baby's body is safe.

Like many of our study participants, Cassie and Thelma spent many hours and invested significant resources – bodily, emotional and financial – to engage in milk sharing. As we discussed in Chapter 2, it is precisely this investment that constitutes the emotional materiality of shared milk. In Chapter 3, we explored the ways our participants became members of milk sharing bio-communities of practice. In this chapter, we focus on the practices of sharing milk that take place within the bio-communities. Specifically, we consider how milk travels from the bodies of donors to those of recipients and how this journey serves to constitute and maintain the bio-communities of practice.

Making milk

At the centre of milk-sharing bio-communities of practice is milk. Making milk is a labour-intensive process that involves unremitting discipline and continual, sustained commitment. Similar to other forms of household and childrearing labour delegated to women in traditional white, heteropatriarchal arrangements (Friedan 1963[2001]; Oakley 1974[2019], 2018; Hochschild 1989), the labour of making milk is obscured by popular representations that erase the work involved and the public/private distinction that relegates it to the home. Notions of breastfeeding as 'natural' suggest that it happens automatically and without any effort, learning, or practice (Locke 2009), and public aversion toward breastfeeding in public relegates such labour to the home, making it hidden and therefore invisible (Stearns 2009). Researchers examining the labour involved in breastfeeding have identified that breastfeeding involves significant bodily labour (Avishai 2004, 2007, 2011; Stearns 2009, 2013), encompassing both 'body work' – work that is done to control, manage, or modify the body – and 'embodied labour' – work that occurs from within the body. In her interviews with mothers who breastfed, Cindy Stearns (2009, 2013) notes that her participants engaged in bodily labour to influence the quality of their milk by controlling the food and substances they consumed and avoiding exposure to chemical toxins. They made efforts to feed and hydrate their bodies to ensure that they could produce enough milk, and they restricted their diets based on perceptions of their children's sensitivities to their milk when they ate certain foods. Similarly, Orit Avishai (2007, 2011) conceptualizes the lactating body as a site of careful management, that her predominantly white, middle-class participants approached much like an exercise regimen by setting goals, measuring output and adhering to strict routines. This embodied labour of breastfeeding is understood to foster production of the highest quality milk at the quantity necessary for feeding one's infant.

Mothers who become breastmilk donors engage in the same bodily labour as mothers who breastfeed their own babies, yet they perform additional work to create milk to give. The labour and self-sacrifice involved in producing milk that becomes shared is part of what makes the milk so special (Shaw 2015, 2019; Falls 2017; Shaw and Morgan 2017; Wilson 2018), contributing to its emotive value. The work is also foundational to milk-sharing bio-communities of practice, as the bio-communities could not exist without the practices – the labour – that constitute them.

Body work

All donors in our study engaged in significant body work to influence the quality of their milk. They carefully monitored intake of foods and substances believed to enhance the quality of breastmilk and restricted those understood to have a detrimental effect. Several donors continued taking prenatal vitamins, and some took other supplements to enhance the healthiness of their breastmilk. They focused on eating healthy foods, restricting or altogether avoiding junk food, caffeine, alcohol and medications, and some avoided foods that they believed produced discomfort in the babies who consumed their milk, such as dairy products, spicy foods, or certain vegetables such as broccoli. Donors also used several tactics to manipulate the quantity of breastmilk they produced. Most took measures to ensure they consumed enough calories and stayed hydrated to support milk production. Some made sure to eat enough fibre or enough fat, whereas others focused on consuming foods that are understood to increase breastmilk production such as oatmeal and flaxseed. A few took the herbal supplement fenugreek and two took the prescription medication Domperidone.

Some donors, such as Elaine, Raven, and Lindsey, took a relaxed approach to managing their milk's quality by limiting intake of junk food, caffeine, or alcohol, but not eliminating it altogether. Elaine, who donated to two recipients, explained:

> 'I took prenatal vitamins when I could remember to take them. Second kid around, you have a hard time remembering stuff. There's some days I didn't even brush my teeth, let alone remember to take the prenatal [she laughs]. I toyed a little bit with taking fenugreek. I took fenugreek with my [first] son, and I did a couple times with her, but honestly I was just so sleep deprived and braindead, I couldn't even remember to take the prenatal, so I didn't really take the fenugreek but maybe a couple of times. So, mostly it was just drinking water and trying to eat healthy. That was about it. And making sure I had high fibre. I mean, the more fibre you have the better your milk production is. I also avoided copious amounts of caffeine. I would have a couple of beers a week, usually on the weekends, but I didn't drink excessively. I didn't drink excessive amounts of caffeine. I avoided diet soda. I avoided all sodas. That was pretty much it.'

On the other end of the spectrum, participants like Christine, Isabella and Georgianna described strict adherence to dietary and lifestyle regimes to ensure their breastmilk was as healthy as possible. This was part of a broader lifestyle that involved extensive labour to attempt to limit exposure to toxins to manage their 'chemical burden' (Mackendrick 2014), and a commitment to 'natural' living through vaccine and medication refusal (Reich 2016). For example, Christine received milk from 40 donors for her foster child and had donated to two recipients at the time of her interview with Beatriz. When asked if she did anything to affect the quality of her milk, Christine explained:

> 'I eat 100% organic. I try to make everything from scratch. We try not to have any processed foods. We don't use any chemical cleaners in the house. I don't and none of my kids have ever had any pharmaceuticals, we don't own any

> Tylenol, Advil, no medicines whatsoever. We use essential oils for pretty much everything. Anything that's come up so far, we've been able to use oils for. So, I try to be completely toxin- and chemical-free. Supplements, I do take fish oil, some Vitamin D, some different things like that.'

Christine described the ways she managed her own health and the quality of her milk in absolute terms, by eating "100% organic", not owning *any* chemical cleaners, and using "no medicines whatsoever". Her strict adherence to these lifestyle regimens is an effort not only to control her own health, but to manage the quality of the breastmilk produced within her body. This form of body work, in the way that Christine enacts it, requires strict self-discipline, and extensive time and effort, as it requires her to cook "everything from scratch".

Several donors eliminated foods from their diets that they thought their own babies were sensitive to, but few eliminated foods solely for peer recipients. Raven, who donated to 12 recipients, described feeling guilty for not eliminating dairy products from her diet for her friend's baby. She explained:

> 'There was this other mom, I really wanted to help her, but she needed dairy-free milk. And I was like, "I can't. I don't have a dairy-free lifestyle." If it was for my own baby, sure I could go dairy-free, but for someone else's baby, that's a huge sacrifice to make. So, I gave her some other resources to maybe try and find some breastmilk that was dairy-free, but I mean, I couldn't help her.'

In other instances, donors indicated their food intake on the milk bags to allow recipient parents to make informed choices about their babies' consumption and to monitor whether or not certain foods had an effect. Hope donated milk to two recipients. She explained that she would distinguish bags of milk that she created after "sipping on a beer" by putting a black dot on them. She continued:

> 'And then I have to keep track for her daughter, because like, "What is your daughter allergic to? What is she sensitive to?" She is like, "You can pretty much eat anything, but the only thing she is sensitive to is broccoli and a few other greens that would make her gassy." So, I am like, "Okay, now I have got to label those ones." I am like, "There is broccoli in this one." … And then she is like, "She does

> kind of have a sensitivity to seafood." I am like, "You are asking the wrong girl to do this right now." So, whenever there is seafood, I try to label it when I remember to do it. And then there are other times I am like, "There is a possibility one of these is not marked and it has broccoli in it and if she is gassy it is not my fault!" [she laughs].'

Like Elaine, Hope's narrative emphasizes that the labour involved in being a milk donor takes place in the midst of mothering young children – a time when many are sleep-deprived and overwhelmed by the labour involved in caregiving (Tomori 2016; Tomori and Boyer 2019).

This work that donors perform to alter their own bodies in order to produce milk that is of high quality and in sufficient quantity to donate is foundational to the emotive value of peer-shared milk. It is the personal sacrifice involved in restricting one's consumption and managing toxic exposure that makes this type of bodily gift unique and special. Whereas other forms of bodily gifts such as blood and banked milk become valuable through their transformation through technological processing (Waldby and Mitchell 2006; Carroll 2014), peer-shared milk becomes valuable, in part, through the bodily processing that occurs as donors control what they consume as a way of manipulating the milk they produce. However, once milk is produced within the body, donors need some way of transferring it to recipients. This occurs through the embodied labour of milk expression – most often pumping – and direct co-feeding.

Embodied labour

The breast pump revolutionized breastfeeding and wet nursing by facilitating the expression of human milk from a woman's body so that it could be fed to a baby through a bottle, allowing the disentanglement of breastmilk feeding and breastfeeding (Bar-Yam 2010; Boyer and Boswell-Penc 2010). However, pumping is hard work that is often described as one of the most uncomfortable and unpleasant aspects of breastfeeding. It is a significant component of the work of breastfeeding (Avishai 2004; Stearns 2009, 2010; Johnson and Salpini 2017; Johnson 2019), and the ability to pump with few obstacles is a common characteristic of breastmilk donors (Osbaldiston and Mingle 2007), whereas difficulty expressing milk and feelings of displeasure while pumping are common reasons mothers trying to breastfeed need to supplement with formula or donor milk (Avishai 2004; Kelleher

2006). Not surprisingly, pumping is conceptualized as a complex and contradictory practice in the social science literature. On one hand, pumping affords some mothers the ability to provide breastmilk to their children while engaging in the paid labour force. This can facilitate work–family balance for some mothers under certain working conditions where time, space and privacy are afforded and problems with breastfeeding or pumping do not emerge (Johnson and Salpini 2017; Porter 2018; Johnson 2019). Pumping may also enable mothers who breastfeed to have a break from their children to engage in adult-centred social life, and provide opportunities for fathers to be involved in feeding (Avishai 2004; Ryan et al 2013; Team and Ryan 2014). On the other hand, scholars also argue that breast pumping contributes to the medicalization and technologizing of breastfeeding, as it facilitates measuring, examining and testing breastmilk, and encourages the consumption of a variety of commercial goods and services that may otherwise be unnecessary (Van Esterik 1996; Stearns 2010; Ryan et al 2013; Afflerback et al 2014; Torres 2014; Porter 2018). Kath Ryan and colleagues (2013) argue that the increasing trend toward pumping commodifies breastmilk, valuing product over process, and diminishes mother–infant bonding by removing the physical contact required for direct breastfeeding.

Social scientists who study breastmilk donation to milk banks recognize milk expression as a significant component of the work of donating milk. Katherine Carroll (2015) conceptualizes donation to milk banks as 'care work', positing that pumping and handling milk is part of the care work milk donors perform. She suggests that this care work supports milk bank donors' identities as 'good mothers' since their labour is consistent with hegemonic ideals of intensive mothering. Similar patterns are identified among peer breastmilk donors, in which the labour and self-sacrifice involved in producing and expressing milk supports mothers' moral identities (Shaw 2015, 2019; Shaw and Morgan 2017; Carter et al 2018; Reyes-Foster and Carter 2018b).

For occasional donors in our study who gave whatever expressed breastmilk they had extra, the embodied labour of producing and expressing breastmilk to give was the same labour they were already performing for their own babies. They expressed milk with the intention of feeding it to their own children and ended up having extra that they donated. For routine donors who pumped specifically for donation, the embodied labour of expressing enough milk to give was typically performed more frequently and involved initiation of a pumping routine designed specifically for expressing excess. For most routine donors, this involved altering how they fed their own babies.

Jane, a routine donor who was also a CLC, donated a few thousand ounces of milk, pumping about a hundred ounces a week for donation. She described pumping as "soooo much work", explaining that "after a while, you just get worn out" from it. Nevertheless, she continued to pump every day to maintain her milk supply and express it for donation. She described her morning routine:

> 'I can pump while I'm battling off the baby and drinking my coffee, but it's harder to get everything done. So literally, I wake up in the morning, I nurse on one side all night, pump the other side in the morning, and then I just keep it in the fridge and store it every couple days.'

To sustain her level of breastmilk donation, Jane altered how she fed Sadie, her own baby. Rather than feeding Sadie from each breast during the night, which would maintain even milk supply and empty each breast, she would feed only from one breast, signalling to her body to continue producing milk. This way, the breast she used to feed Sadie would produce enough milk to keep her nourished, while the other breast would produce excess milk that can be donated. Each morning, Jane pumped whichever breast was full of milk, and later prepared the pumped milk for donation.

Jane's milk expression routine demonstrates the interembodied nature of peer breastmilk sharing. She altered the way she fed Sadie as a way of encouraging her body to produce extra milk that she could donate. This not only modifies her own body, by increasing the amount of milk it produces, but it potentially modifies Sadie's body by altering the milk she receives at night. Current knowledge of breastmilk suggests that the milk changes in composition as it is released from the breast throughout a feeding, with the early milk being thinner and less fatty (referred to as 'foremilk'), and the later milk being thicker and more fatty (referred to as 'hindmilk'). Some experts argue that the foremilk/hindmilk dichotomy is an oversimplification, but most agree that breastmilk changes in its composition the longer the child is at the breast (Ballard and Morrow 2013). By feeding Sadie only from one breast all night long, Jane could be altering the composition of the milk Sadie receives, thereby modifying her body. In addition, breastmilk is understood to be produced to meet the baby's demand, so Sadie continuing to 'demand' more milk from the same breast all night stimulates Jane's body to continue producing milk. In this way, the embodied labour she engages in to maintain excess milk to donate involves the interembodiment of herself and her baby – an element of breastfeeding identified in the social science literature (Ryan et al. 2011; Lupton 2013).

As Jane continued her milk-sharing story, she described the challenges of caring for her two children while pumping each morning. Although the question was about safety precautions, her response highlights the labour involved in managing Sadie while engaging in the embodied labour of pumping.

> 'In interest of fairness, I also have a baby on my lap who's trying to grab at the pump and grab at the tubing and stuff as I'm pumping. So, it's not a sterile process, but it doesn't really have to be. If it had to be, I would make that happen, but it's breastmilk, it doesn't need to be.'

Several donors provided similar descriptions of difficulties involved in caring for their own babies while simultaneously pumping for donation. Most babies did not appear to enjoy their mothers' pumping, often becoming territorial over their milk. This made pumping – a task that is already described as unpleasant under the best conditions – even more challenging while simultaneously caring for one's own baby. Hope summarized: "God forbid if I bring out the pump my daughter wants to break it. She will take it and go, 'No milky, my boobies.'"

This jealousy among babies and sense of ownership of their mother's milk was even more apparent when donors gave milk directly from their breast through co-feeding. To soothe their own babies while breastfeeding a recipient baby, donors who co-fed would often breastfeed both children at the same time, commonly referred to as 'tandem nursing'. Tandem nursing involves the interembodiment of the donor, the donor's baby, and the recipient baby, who experience shared breastfeeding together. Jane described her co-feeding experience:

> 'Essentially, I just nursed a friend's child when I watched him. Because he was a toddler at the time and I was watching him and he just had an epic meltdown. So, I called my friend and she was too far away and she begged me to nurse him so I did. So, I definitely have a respect for wet nursing, and I would definitely do it again if the situation was necessary. I certainly wouldn't have an issue with somebody doing it for my child if the situation were necessary as well. But the experience was weird. Every baby latches differently, plus it was a toddler. So, it wasn't this sweet little helpless baby, it was this toddler. And then

> my toddler came up and wanted to nurse too, and then they were poking at each other while they were nursing. It was definitely a strange experience.... I don't know that it would have been quite so strange if he had been a baby. I mean this was a whole person that had a personality and everything, you know? Babies are kind of a bit different. It's, like I said, it was just the whole, two toddlers up there and poking at each other and I was just – it was definitely weird but it wasn't bad. It was just an interesting experience.'

The episode Jane described highlights the interactions between the three individuals involved in her co-feeding experience that shaped the situation. As she fed her friend's toddler, Sam, and her own toddler, Avery, one at each breast, and they latched on and drew milk from her, they also interacted with one another. The embodied labour of co-feeding extended beyond the dyadic interembodiment of the donating mother and the recipient child, to include the donating mother's own child as well. This was a common theme among donors who engaged in co-feeding. In tandem co-feeding – where a mother simultaneously breastfeeds her own child and a recipient child – the mother's embodied labour involves not only the interembodiment of breastfeeding the two children at the same time, but also the disciplinary role of managing the children's interactions with one another. The tandem co-feeding situation typically arises out of the mother's attempts at 'emotion work' (Hochschild 1983, 1989) to manage her own child's feelings about her breastfeeding an unrelated child. The child's sense of possessiveness over the mother's milk – or at least the mothers' perceptions of it – speaks to the emotional materiality of milk, or the sense that the milk is something more than just a fluid containing nutrients and immunoglobulins, but that it is a container of human connection, emotion and, most of all, love.

Managing the inventory

For donors who gave expressed milk, handling and storing milk was a significant and time-consuming component of the practice of milk sharing. The ABM (2010) has established protocols for handling and storing breastmilk for home use for full-term infants that recommend washing hands before expressing milk, washing or sanitizing containers and pumping equipment before use, storing milk for no more than eight hours (refrigerator) or six months (freezer), and transporting milk on ice. Although all participants worked to manage, store and transport milk safely, most but not all followed the ABM guidelines. In analyzing our online survey data, we found that 73.8% of peer milk donors reported 'always' or 'often' engaging in at least four of the ABM safety guidelines (Reyes-Foster et al 2017). The practice most commonly circumvented was transporting milk on ice. Most participants transferred milk locally and in person, and while they took measures to ensure the milk stayed frozen during transportation, by packing it in a cooler or insulated bag, they did not always use ice.

Donors described routines they employed for handling and storing their milk and described spaces and 'stations' they set up to facilitate their practices. Lisa told Shannon her milk-sharing story outside at a coffee shop near the beach on a sunny September morning. She explained that she typically washes her hands before pumping, except for her 3.00 am pump, which she did religiously for the first four months of her child, Mason's, life. She described her middle-of-the-night routine:

> 'For the 3.00 am feedings, I have hand sanitizer by the bed because he co-slept and it's easier that way, rather than getting out of bed all the time. I'm scared to death that he's going to fall off the bed all the time. I have the pump and the bottle on my night stand, him in the bed, dog at the foot of the bed, pump, and sanitizer.'

Curious about how she handled the milk once it was pumped since she seemed to avoid leaving Mason in the bed, Shannon asked, "Did you get up to put the milk away or did you wait until morning?" Lisa responded:

> 'Oh yeah, I would first check on Mason, put pillows around him, then get up, go tiptoe into the kitchen, pour the milk into the bag, date it and write the ounces, put it in the freezer. Then I would have a little tally of how many ounces I had, at the top.'

She continued, describing the station she set up with her milk storage supplies:

> 'I have my cabinet, it has my pump in there and my bottles, and underneath that is my microwave. But right in between that and the wall are my bags, and right above that is a little Sharpie [marker pen] on a string.... It's really easy, so

> I have my pump and my bottles and you know, I put it all together, and it goes into the bag, everything goes into the sink to get cleaned. And I put the ounces and the number on it, and it goes into my little cardboard thing that holds the bags of milk in the freezer. Then the pump gets cleaned and I sterilize it while he's asleep.'

Even in the middle of the night, donors followed routines that helped ensure the cleanliness and safety of their expressed milk.

Donors often took great care to portion their milk to facilitate thawing and feeding (see Figure 4.1) and minimize waste. Elaine described her very intricate method for portioning her milk:

> 'It automatically went into breastmilk collection bags, and then into the freezer.... I would have the milk in the collection bottles. When I would finish it all up, I would put the breast pump parts into the sink to be washed. I'd have the bottles there, I'd portion it out in four-ounce servings – all my milk was always in four-ounce servings. Then four ounces would go into the bag, it would be labelled and dated, and I would write how much – sometimes it was four-and-a-half ounces. If I had maybe two ounces left over, then that would go into the fridge, and then that would go into the freezer with the next time I had another two ounces. So I froze in equal four ounce portions into the bags. I have a flat, small cookie sheet in the freezer so then I would lay the bags flat to freeze, they froze faster that way. And then I would put, then I would have a large, gallon, freezer Ziploc bag that would be labelled from the dates, from, you know, December 1st to December 5th, and I would put in 12 servings from that period of time, and then I would save them in dozen bags. And so then in the back freezer – I have a back chest freezer – then I would have the milk separated into dozen portions. You know, and each bag of a dozen has four-ounce portions.'

Elaine's narrative depicts the very detailed and precise method of measuring, managing and storing her breastmilk once it was pumped. She followed the explanation with a chuckle and added, "My mom's a nurse. I got a little anal on that side of the process." This attention to detail, with the establishment and maintenance of a methodical routine and a station to facilitate it, was common among donors.

Figure 4.1: Milk storage and organization

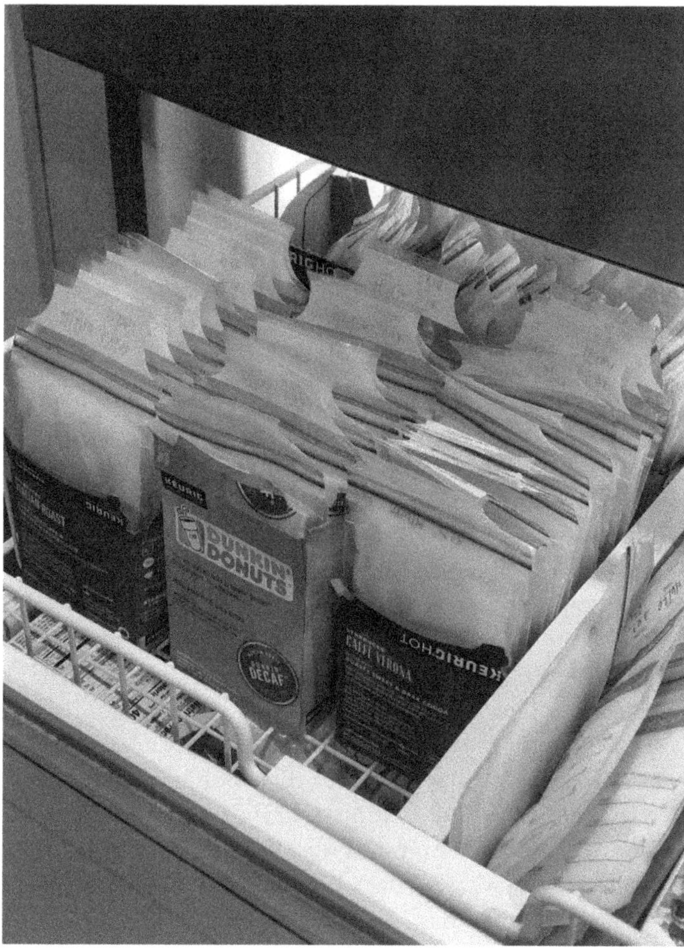

Source: Courtesy of Brittany Durrani

Finding each other

For milk sharing to take place, donors and recipients must find each other, and both parties need to agree that they want to participate in transferring milk. This process, what Tanya Cassidy (2012a) calls 'making milky matches', entails navigating milk-sharing communities to establish connections between an individual who has milk to give and one who wishes to receive it. Donors and recipients find each other through various paths, ranging from existing close relationships, to connections through broader online and offline social networks, to public posts on the internet. The social forces and mediums of communication that bring them together are connected to the paths that lead them to become donors and recipients in the first place, and their relationships and connections to milk-sharing bio-communities of practice, as well as the broader communities that support them.

For a milky match to occur, a donor and recipient need to recognize each other as a potential match. Donors found it relatively easy to find potential milk recipients, but for most recipients, identifying potential donors was an ongoing, time-consuming, and emotionally taxing endeavour. Most had multiple donors, sometimes as many as 40 or 50, with the median being eight. Those who received milk from multiple donors utilized several methods to find and screen them. Although their methods were often informal, the screening procedures recipients used guided their decisions to decline milk on occasion, with 28% (N=40) of recipients who took our survey declining milk at least once.

Christine was pregnant with her first child when she became a foster mother to baby Liam. Because she was not producing any breastmilk of her own, she continuously sought out donors. She explained:

> 'So, we took him in, and he was young, about eight months. And I wanted to be able to give him breastmilk instead of formula. And so, I started looking around to find breastmilk, and I started getting it from my midwife, from my doctor, from Human Milk 4 Human Babies Facebook page, Eats on Feets, and I ended up getting 6,000 ounces for him total. I was able to keep him on breastmilk until his one-year adjusted age, and then even after that he was able to get one bottle of breastmilk every day until he was two.'

Later in the interview, Christine explained her process for identifying donors, starting with those closest in her social network and slowly moving outward. When asked how she typically found donors, she explained:

> 'Word of mouth. With my friends, all of my friends breastfeed, pretty much, so all of them would give me extra if they had any. I asked my chiropractor and my midwife, because my midwife was in touch, her patient had lost her baby right after she was born, and she'd already been pumping a lot, and so all the milk went to me. And my midwife actually pumped milk for me. She was still breastfeeding, and so she had some extra milk saved up that

she gave to me during the process as well. So, between my chiropractor and my midwife, they spread the word around that I needed milk. And so a lot of the milk came from them, and when that wasn't enough, I would post in the breastfeeding support groups asking for milk, and when that was not enough, I would look in Human Milk 4 Human Babies and Eats on Feets Facebook groups.'

Christine's process of identifying donors illustrates a common pattern, where donors and recipients began searching for matches within their close social networks, expanding out as needed. Many, particularly those who had established connections or were integrated in the broader communities that supported milk sharing, found matches through friends and family.

One such participant is Ingrid, who donated milk to ten recipients. As she recounted her milk-sharing experience to Beatriz, she explained how she identified recipients:

> 'I think it's all mutual friends. I don't think I've found anyone – just, my sister is like, "Hey, I have a mom in need." And then, her friend in Georgia that we drove to, they've been friends since middle school, and then another girl that I donated a lot to. Most of my recipients are long-term recipients. Their babies are totally fed off of my milk, so they are not getting anything else but my milk. So the little girl that was failure to thrive, she was totally fed off my milk for the first year. And I had another friend from my church. So, yeah, they've all been long term – most of them have been long term. So, that's how I've, like, my first donation to my friend with the failure-to-thrive baby, the first donation I gave her was 700 ounces. And then I had another friend who, at four months I met her through a mutual friend at church and started donating to her daughter. She was like, "I have this friend. Her baby can't tolerate formula, and she's only ten pounds. She's three months." She knew that I was looking for someone to give my milk to because I had so much.'

When asked if she did anything to screen recipients, Ingrid continued:

> 'No, I don't screen them. I meet them and I meet their babies, and make sure they have babies, and they're not using

> the milk for weird things. And, I have a list of blood work that I give if they want it. I tell them all the medications that I take. I just take prenatal vitamins, and we eat organic. So, I give them a list of my blood work if they want it, and most of the time they don't because they know me. But I have it available.'

Like other donors and recipients, Ingrid identified all of her matches through friends and family. She was integrated in social networks of mothers who valued breastmilk feeding, making it easy for her to identify recipients. She developed long-term milk-sharing relationships with many of them, which meant she did not have to look further for additional recipients.

Some donors and recipients identified matches through their local community networks, using online social networking sites to facilitate connections. These participants were integrated in local networks of mothers who were committed to breastfeeding, and where breastmilk sharing could be facilitated. They identified recipients who were their friends, acquaintances, or were recognizable through private Facebook groups that centred on aspects of mothering related to breastfeeding and natural parenting but were not established to facilitate milk sharing. From our survey sample, 42.4% of participants reported using local private Facebook groups (local breastfeeding or parenting groups) to identify donors or recipients, with 12.3% using their own Facebook pages (Reyes-Foster et al 2015). Typically, when donors and recipients were connected through mutual friends or smaller online networks, screening procedures tended to be informal, although some donors provided their most recent bloodwork.

Nicole, who gave milk to five recipients, used private Facebook groups centred on breastfeeding and natural parenting to identify recipients who were connected to her broader social network. When asked how she identified recipients, she answered:

> 'All through Facebook groups. Our local Lactating Mamas group and another one that's for Volusia County that's called Volusia Moms Network. And then another, the last person that I've been donating to is my babysitter. She's wet nursing a foster baby for her parents. And, so I'm donating to them to use at night.... So, most of them are friends of friends, or I actually know the person, so I've never donated to anybody that I didn't personally know or didn't know somebody that knew them.'

Some donors and recipients were matched through a third party, such as Get Pumped, a local birth centre, or a 'peer broker', often a mutual friend who would collect milk from a donor and distribute it to a recipient. This form of distribution eliminated the need for participants to identify matches on their own, but it required a certain level of integration in the social networks to know about Get Pumped or to be connected with midwives or peer brokers who would facilitate for them. Get Pumped also has a formal screening process that includes a health questionnaire and blood test that donors are required to complete before their milk is accepted. The organization has several drop-off sites throughout Central Florida and organized an annual social picnic that provided opportunities for donors and recipients to meet. Two of our interviewees brought their milk to a drop-off location with the intention of donating it to Get Pumped and met a potential recipient in the process. Raven, who had donated exclusively to Get Pumped, told Shannon the story of how she met Mona Lisa, her first and only direct recipient:

> 'I went to my chiropractor's office and I was dropping off milk for Get Pumped. And there was a mom there, Mona Lisa, with her baby and I guess she overheard me talking about how much milk I had and her baby was lactose intolerant and she didn't make enough milk to feed to her baby and so she couldn't have formula either and her baby was really sick. And she was like, "Can I just have some of your milk?" And I was like, "Sure. Go ahead, have my milk." Like you can't, a mom can't sit there with her sick baby and look at you and ask, "Can I have some?" and you say "No." I mean, you're gonna say yes! So, I gave half to her and half to Get Pumped. I gave her 100 and some ounces and 100 and some ounces to Get Pumped that donation.'

Like Raven, most participants who donated milk through a third party also gave directly to recipients, at least once, and none of our recipients received milk exclusively from a formal organization or healthcare provider. Instead, these platforms were used for many as one of several methods to identify matches. Sometimes a donor–recipient pair would initially be connected through a third party and would then continue their milk-sharing relationship on their own.

As seen in Christine's story, when all other approaches were exhausted, participants would seek local matches through the public Facebook pages of milk-sharing organizations like Eats on Feets or

Human Milk 4 Human Babies. For most recipients in our study, this method was a 'last resort' since it connected them with individuals outside their extended social networks, and recipients utilized a stricter set of measures to screen potential donors they met on these sites than for those identified through their own networks. For donors in our study, these sites provided an opportunity for those who were less integrated in the milk-sharing networks to establish connections and create their own communities (Figure 4.2). Although they started out as strangers, many participants developed long-term milk-sharing relationships with matches identified through these websites, and some formed close friendships.

Figure 4.2: Human Milk 4 Human Babies Facebook post

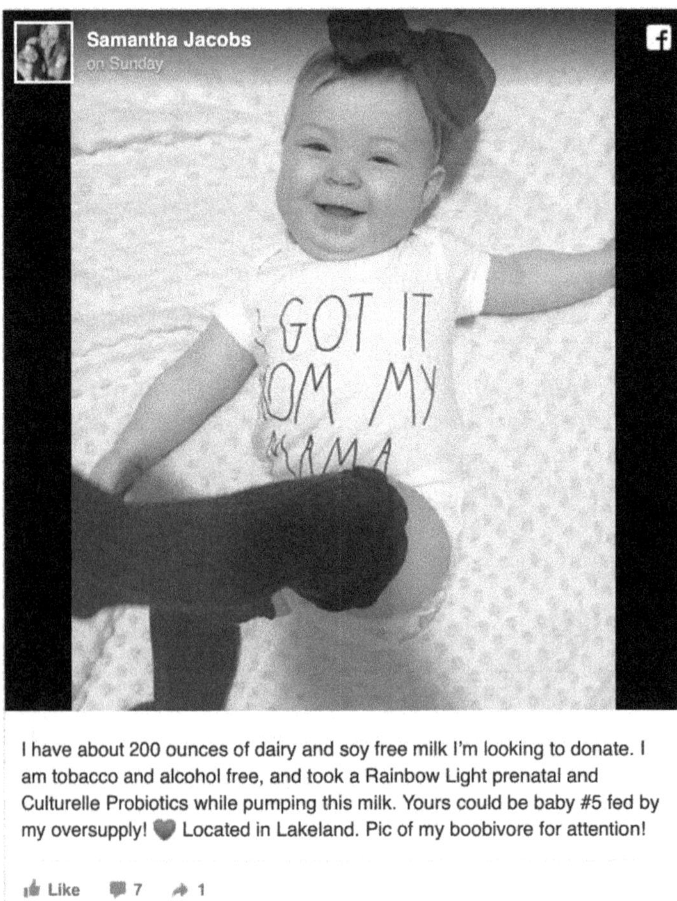
Samantha Jacobs
on Sunday
GOT IT
I have about 200 ounces of dairy and soy free milk I'm looking to donate. I am tobacco and alcohol free, and took a Rainbow Light prenatal and Culturelle Probiotics while pumping this milk. Yours could be baby #5 fed by my oversupply! Located in Lakeland. Pic of my boobivore for attention!
Like 7 1

Source: Courtesy of Samantha Jacobs

Although she received milk from many donors within her network, the internet played an important role in Christine's ability to procure milk. She met a handful of donors through public milk-sharing sites, and one whom she met through Human Milk 4 Human Babies pumped milk for her every day, donating a couple of thousand ounces just to Christine. She explained the variability in the amount of milk she had on hand at any given time, and described her process of finding more when she ran low:

> 'I made it a goal to never give him a drop of formula, so I was very busy going to get all the milk. Because there would be mornings where I would wake up and I would have one bag of milk left in the freezer, and I would know he needs, you know, six bottles that day. So, I would just pray and pray, "Please send some milk, please, please, please." I'd go through all my contacts, "Anybody got any?" And like, there was twice where he drank his last bag, and then we had to go drive and pick up his next. So, there were times where my freezer was full, and there were times where I was frantically looking for it. So, I spent a lot of time getting it all. And if I had a lot of other children, I don't know that I could have spent that much time. Because I'm in Altamonte, a lot of the milk was coming from Deltona, from all over, and so it was a whole, whole lot of driving. And then sometimes moms would tell me that they had milk, like in the example of my regular donor, her freezer defrosted one weekend and she lost over 600 ounces from her deep freezer defrosting. And so, I would take a setback. Many times, I would be expecting to get milk and then suddenly I wouldn't have any. So, between all the 40 donors, I was having to regularly stay in touch with who had milk and who didn't and trying to find it.'

For Christine and other recipients, finding enough donors to exclusively feed breastmilk was a stressful process that required extensive effort and persistent dedication. When individual social circles were insufficient at providing enough milk, public Facebook sites became important resources for connecting individuals who were searching for a match.

Facebook was also a forum where donors and recipients screened each other to determine whether or not they were compatible. Some recipients, like Christine, relied on their knowledge of potential donors' lifestyles when receiving milk through their extended social networks, but requested bloodwork from donors they met online. Others, like Thelma, relied more heavily on people's Facebook profiles than on bloodwork. Thelma explained:

> 'I don't do any medical screening, test-wise. Because I feel like you can have screenings two months ago and the status today could be completely different. You could have screenings at the beginning of your pregnancy and nine months later your screening could be completely different. So, I don't do medical screenings. I just talk to them, talk about medications, drugs, alcohol, any concerns. I like to meet their babies because if they are nursing their healthy babies then I know their milk is healthy because they're not going to be nursing their babies if it's going to kill their baby, you know. So, meeting healthy babies is really important to me.... And you can learn a lot about someone through their Facebook profile. *A lot* about someone. So, I always Facebook stalk them as well. I always add them as a friend and if they deny it, that's an immediate red flag to me. You know, if you are wanting to share milk with my baby and you won't even accept my friend request on Facebook? But, if they accept my friend request, I usually go back three years' worth or whatever, just scrolling. This is part of my screening. I am sure they're doing the same to my profile too.'

Thelma was right that screening happened on both sides. Although most donors only turned down direct requests for milk when they did not have enough to give, and most could not think of any other scenarios where they would decline giving milk, they still screened potential recipients, especially when considering requests on Facebook. As other scholars have noted (Falls 2017; Wilson 2018), there is often a hierarchy of recipients who are most desired by donors, where babies who are adopted, suffer from a health condition, or are younger are prioritized over others. Thus, recipients felt they had to make a compelling case for why they should be selected to receive a donor's milk. Thelma moved to Florida while receiving peer milk for her son William, eventually becoming an administrator of a public milk-sharing Facebook page. Spending extensive time on the page, she knew the kinds of requests for milk that received a response, and, as a result, provided detailed information in her posts.

When Beatriz asked if she ever felt that she was screened by donors, Thelma responded:

> 'Oh yes. *Oh yes.* Especially as your baby gets older. I've noticed being on the admin side that mothers that have a very brief, "I need milk, I'm located in Orlando," they don't get responses. It's just because, well, "Why do you need milk? How old is your baby? What is your baby's name?" And they just don't share the information. "Why aren't you producing milk?" So, I felt like I always shared my story, you know. I would type up a new one every single time I messaged someone to make it personal. I would never copy and paste because it just didn't feel right to me because milk sharing is really personal. So, I would share our story, maybe his age, his name, I would usually send a picture. And occasionally, as he got older people would stop replying, but I would notice when he was younger everyone replied, even if it was, "I already found a mom, thank you, good luck." But as a he got older people would just stop replying. It was like, well, okay, it's obviously just how it works. When your baby is older people don't want to share milk with you, that's okay.'

Thelma highlighted the common view that sharing milk is an intimate, personal endeavour, which makes asking for breastmilk a significant social encounter. By watching patterns of interactions on Facebook, observing which posts are successful, she figured out how to achieve the greatest response.

For some recipients, asking for milk was an emotionally troubling aspect of milk sharing. Shirley, who worked as a birth doula and peer lactation counsellor, experienced low milk supply with both of her children despite her knowledge and experience helping other women breastfeed. Her midwife provided her with the phone number for another mother, Sara, who was known to be actively donating, to call for potential milk. Shirley described how it felt to ask Sara for milk:

> 'To me it feels like asking for money, asking for donor milk. It feels almost like asking someone for money. It's like asking for a handout to feed my kid and that's really hard. I don't, I don't know why it feels that way, but it does.'

In a social context where self-sufficiency and independence are highly valued, it is not surprising that many recipients – who were predominantly white and class-privileged – were uncomfortable asking for milk. For some, like Shirley, coming to terms with their inability to provide enough milk and asking for help were deeply humbling experiences.

Transferring

The transfer of milk from donor to recipient was an important social encounter that entailed not only attending to safety measures such as screening and safe handling, but also provided opportunities for the development of trust, friendship and community. Consistent with other social science research on the practice of milk sharing (Thorley 2012; Palmquist and Doehler 2016; Falls 2017; Wilson 2018), most donors and recipients met in person to transfer milk. Of the 168 donors who took our online survey (Reyes-Foster et al 2015), only 5.95% (N=10) reported *ever* transferring milk by mail. Most commonly (68.45%, N=115), donors personally delivered their milk, had it picked up directly by a recipient, or met recipients in a public location. The remaining participants (23.21%, N=39) handed their milk to a mediator who delivered it to the recipient, or dropped it off at a third-party location (such as a birth centre or Get Pumped drop-off point) (2.38%, N=4). Among recipients, only 6.5% (N=12) in our survey, and none whom we interviewed, ever received milk by mail.

Most recipients considered meeting in person an important part of the screening process. Thelma, who identified many of her donors through Eats on Feets, emphasized the importance of meeting to transfer milk.

> 'It's very important to meet face to face. It's very important to me. I feel like it's just the basics of safe milk sharing is meeting, sharing your expectations, having a connection with the mother. I have turned down milk before based on meeting the donor. I just wasn't comfortable with this mom. I just didn't, it was something about her. I didn't like it. It didn't feel right. I feel like, I have always felt like it was good, you know. And meeting a mom was always, even when it was a first-time donation for the mom, it's always a little bit awkward. And the people who have donated multiple times are usually a little bit more comfortable. So

> even those awkward situations, it wasn't anything like that, it just didn't – I think it was just a combination of how she acted and maybe just a gut response.'

As Thelma hesitated, Beatriz assured her that we were not judging her, but just wanted to understand. When asked what kind of things might have set off warning signals, Thelma sighed and admitted:

> 'Cleanliness, hygiene. I don't know, without sounding like a horrible person – the way they carry themselves, the way they talk. If you can't figure out how to put two words together, you know, appropriately, then I am a little concerned. So, we have turned down offers before. From one mom, even after I had said, you know, that I wasn't comfortable she insisted that we take her milk. And I took it because she wasn't giving me another option and I threw it away. It was probably 200 ounces, but she wouldn't let me say no. I have no idea why she wouldn't let me say no. She insisted and I said thank you and we parted ways and that was awkward.'

For a few recipients, like Thelma, an in-person transfer generated feelings of discomfort, leading them to decline milk or politely accept it but either discard it or pass it on to someone who was not alarmed by whatever social cues they interpreted as warning signs. In the scenario Thelma described, however reluctantly, she drew on social class markers like speech patterns to interpret her sense of discomfort with milk she was offered. These signs are important to recipients because, unlike most other gifts, breastmilk is a bodily gift. Its quality and purity is presumed to be intricately connected to the characteristics of the individual who produces and gives it, contributing to the importance of meeting in person (Sussman 1982; Shaw 2015, 2019; Shaw and Morgan 2017; Reyes-Foster and Carter 2018a, 2018b).

Meeting in person to transfer milk also created opportunities for the development of trusting relationships, friendship and community, as noted by other milk-sharing scholars (Thorley 2012; Falls 2017; Gribble 2018; Wilson 2018). These characteristics made the milk transfer a special occasion for some donors too. Elaine donated about 1,000 ounces to two recipients whom she met through Human Milk 4 Human Babies. After screening recipients on Facebook by previewing their profiles and scrolling through their baby's photos, and ultimately identifying a recipient, she would invite them to her home to pick up the milk. She explained why this was important to her:

> 'I want to see their baby. I want to meet them face to face. I did invite them to my home. It turned out for one of the ladies it was easier for her to meet me at my workplace, so we met there. This is all a community effort. It's that village mentality. I want to meet you, come over to the house, come meet my children. You know where I live, I get to see your baby.'

For Elaine, giving milk was a significant social encounter, an opportunity to share the intimate space of her home with potential recipients and to meet each other's loved ones. It was about more than just transferring milk from one person to another but provided an occasion to develop interpersonal connections.

By the same token, Cassie described meeting recipients as an emotionally fulfilling aspect of milk sharing. When asked about meeting recipients in person, she exclaimed:

> 'That's the most rewarding part! And like I said, the woman that came up from Tampa, meeting her and talking with her husband and seeing her little baby and holding him and all these things – it was just very fulfilling.'

While meeting in person to transfer milk was typically an interpersonally rewarding aspect of milk sharing, it became taxing over time for long-term participants. For recipients in particular, picking up milk was ongoing and time-consuming, with some driving an hour or longer to get milk. Christine emphasized the time and labour involved in picking up milk, stating that, "If I had a lot of other children, I don't know that I could have spent that much time. It was a whole, whole lot of driving."

Some donors also felt overextended by delivering milk, sometimes dropping recipients as a result. Sara, who donated over 4,000 ounces to more than 30 recipients, including some through Get Pumped, explained:

> 'What I ended up doing is, I was going to a breastfeeding support group every week at Holistic Health Birth Center, and I would just bring a few hundred ounces with me for them to keep my milk there. They would stock their fridge

> with it and give it out to whoever calls and needs it. I've agreed to let my medical information be shared with people, what I'm taking, and things like that. I donate regularly to one person in particular, who, if I don't pump any extra, she gets it first, and then whatever is left over goes to Holistic Health. I used to donate to other moms as well, but I found myself driving everywhere dropping milk off and then I was feeling really thinned out by it. Everybody wanted milk, everybody was desperate for it, and I didn't like having to choose who to give it to. Everyone desperately wants it, everyone desperately needs it. Now I have connected with one mom in particular, she's been the most generous towards me in providing me with all the milk bags I need, so she and I are really close friends now. So, she gets my milk first and whatever is left goes to Holistic Health and they can figure out who needs it most.'

Later in the interview, Sara elaborated on how the transferring of milk became too much work for her.

> 'When I first was donating, a few recipients would just text me when they needed milk. But that was really trying on me because it was constantly like, it felt like people were constantly asking me. I was juggling like four or five at once, so it was a lot. It was constantly like, "I need milk," "No, I need milk," and it could be overwhelming. So finally, I just started to say, "Well, I'll be at Holistic Health on Thursday. You can meet me there." Or I would leave it in Holistic Health's freezer with their name on it. Or the chiropractor that I, we all go to, you know, Dr Leila, she also is a part of Get Pumped. So, there's a lot of places throughout the county that will let me leave my milk in their freezer. And moms have come and picked it up there.'

Although Sara minimized her efforts to deliver milk by dropping it off at a central location, she still, like other donors and recipients throughout our study, carefully prepared her milk to ensure it would stay frozen while in transport.

> 'Normally I'm giving away several hundreds of ounces at once. So, I bag it in hundred ounce – I do have five-ounce milk bags, obviously – and then I put them in a Publix bag

> into hundred-ounce sections or whatever. And then Shirley comes and picks up from my house normally and she just brings a cooler. And they've been in my freezer until they get put in a cooler and then she goes home. When I go to Holistic Health Birth Center, I put them in a cooler and put them right in the freezer as soon as I get there. So, it's usually several hundred ounces, so several Publix bags filled. If it was gonna be longer than – it takes me about 15, 20 minutes to get somewhere. If it was gonna be longer than that then I would probably do something like stuff newspaper and ice packs in the cooler, you know. In order to help keep the cold in longer I would put ice packs and then put newspaper around it to help keep the cold in. The more packed a cooler is, the more insulated it is, the longer it will stay colder. But in general, it's 15 minutes so it doesn't have time to even start to defrost.'

Although many participants, like Sara, did not regularly transport milk on ice, as recommended by the ABM, they took measures to ensure their milk would stay frozen during the transfer from donor to recipient.

Sara's description also highlights the collaboration between local businesses and health providers who facilitate milk sharing by providing freezer space for donors and recipients to use to transfer milk, and sometimes distributing a donor's milk themselves. This came up in our interview with Madeline, a midwife and owner of Holistic Health Birth Center. Madeline confirmed that Holistic Health serves as a drop-off and pick-up point for Get Pumped, but more commonly, they coordinate milk sharing among clients in their office. She explained, "Usually we have them drop it off here and we give it as needed, but if someone needs a long-term donor we will connect them directly and let them figure out what works best for them." These drop-off points eased the burden of transporting milk but removed the interpersonal connections fostered by meeting in person.

Receiving from the breast

Although the transfer of expressed breastmilk is the most common form of peer milk sharing in the Global North, sharing milk through direct feeding (co-feeding) also occurs (Shaw 2007; Thorley 2008, 2009; Wilson 2018). Among our survey participants who ever received milk, 25% (N=38) reported receiving peer milk through co-feeding (Reyes-Foster et al 2015). For some, allowing someone else to breastfeed their child was an emotionally taxing experience. Carmen, a mother of two who took our survey, experienced difficulty breastfeeding her babies. She explained:

> 'My own children were nourished by the milk of generous and kindhearted donors when, despite all the right support, effort, and medication (including Domperidone and herbs) I couldn't produce enough for them.'

Carmen received milk from Get Pumped, as well as from friends and acquaintances, totalling an estimated 20 donors. She described two experiences where her children were co-fed by donors:

> 'My best friend offered while she was visiting, in lieu of supplementing with pumped donor milk. On another occasion, a donor asked if I would mind if she nursed my daughter while she nursed her own rather than preparing a bottle.'

Carmen continued:

> 'It was an emotionally trying experience to let someone else nurse my children, and drove home all the feelings of failure that I had relating to my own supply issues, but I was grateful that people offered and glad to allow it because it helped them feel more connected to the baby they were donating to.'

These feelings of emotional torment from seeing another mother breastfeed one's baby is a reason several recipients were only willing to accept expressed milk. Shirley, who fed her baby Vivian donated milk from Sara through an SNS, explained that she would not want anyone else to experience the level of connection established through breastfeeding. When asked if she would allow Vivian to be co-fed, she responded:

> 'I don't think I could handle it. There's such a connection between me and my daughter and even with all of the plastic that's involved, nursing is still really special. It's like, such a deep bond that I have with her. There's a time of the day, like the witching hour between 9 o'clock and midnight for her where I'm the only one who helps her. She is

> seriously attached to me. She's like, "I smell something good over here." Plus, she's finally getting tired, so she wants to nurse. I have to nurse her to sleep a lot. From 9 o'clock to midnight she cluster-feeds and nurses and she will dry nurse, she doesn't care if there's anything there or not. She wants mommy, and I am the only solution. Daddy cuddling her, giving her a paci [pacifier], walking her around will not work. A bottle won't work. I'm the only solution and it's such a sweet thing, and so nursing for me is such a deep bond with her.'

Not all mothers experienced misgivings or emotional turmoil over having their baby nursed by another person. Thelma benefitted from a large community of women who were willing to nurse her second child, William. Assuming her initial breastfeeding difficulties were a result of a difficult birth, Thelma attempted to exclusively breastfeed her son and "carry on as if I would have a milk supply. But I never did." Thelma's midwife, who supported her desire to have William exclusively breastfed, told her, "Well, you want your baby to be breastfed, so we are going to have your baby breastfed."

Soon, Thelma's house was filled with visiting women ready to nurse baby William. In her interview, Thelma referred to them as wet nurses, even though none of them were paid. She reminisced:

> 'It just started off with all the wet nurses, and my midwife had all her friends coming over, and all her clients coming over, and I would go to them sometimes and we would have events. And you know, we'll be like, "Well, William is hungry, William's hungry, you know who has the fullest boobs?" So, it was like a joke!'

Thelma was ensconced in a community of nursing mothers who were happy to nurse baby William. When she and her husband, who is in the military, received sudden orders to relocate to Central Florida, her friends sent her off with several coolers full of frozen milk and dry ice.

Managing the stash

Just as donors have to create a plan for storing and handling their milk, so, too, do recipients. Once milk is obtained, the work of storing and handling milk can be consuming. One might recall the lengths to which Anna went to ensure not a drop of donor milk went to waste when she was feeding Grace. Like some of our donors, several recipients reported having an additional freezer or deep freezer in their garage that was dedicated primarily to storing breastmilk. Most of the time, recipients used the milk rather quickly, so they did not need to be concerned about expiration dates. However, recipients like Christine who obtained large volumes of milk from scores of peer donors, had to pay greater attention to expiration dates and manage their milk accordingly. Christine explained:

> 'We have a deep freezer. So, all of the milk would go in the deep freezer. And normally I never got a donation big enough that I had to sort it out by date and be concerned about finishing it off. Usually it was, it had just been pumped within the last month or two. So, I wasn't worried about it ever, you know, reaching an expiration date of six or 12 months or whatever. But some of the moms did not find the milk until late. I remember I did get a call from one mom saying, "It hasn't been in a deep freezer, and it's been in there for five-and-a-half months. I've only got a few weeks left technically, if we're going by the six months. Do you want it now?" So there were a few times where I did watch the date, but otherwise, I would pull out what I thought he would need for the day and put it in our regular freezer, and then I would put – I would just take it out and put it in a little water, a little bag of water, and let it defrost, and give him a few ounces at a time, and store the bag in the fridge. If it was a huge bag, like six to ten ounces and he only needed three, I would defrost the whole thing, and pour three ounces in a bottle, and put the three-ounce bag back in the fridge. I would defrost usually about twice a day. So, I would defrost everything I thought he needed for the morning, and then I'd take out the rest and defrost everything I thought he needed for the night. I would defrost it all in room-temperature water.'

As Christine's explanation shows, milk-handling routines not only entailed ensuring proper safety procedures but also estimating just the right amount of milk to make sure none went to waste. She continued:

> 'And, I had to be careful that I would use it all up within the 24 hours, because sometimes there would be a bag hidden in my fridge that I didn't remember I had defrosted

> that morning, or something like that. And so, I had to keep an eye on that.... There were definitely a few times where I missed a bag in the fridge or left something out. One terrible time, there was a Ziploc bag, and I was going through my freezer sorting it to make sure I had enough milk, and I did leave one Ziploc bag out, of milk, and didn't find it until the next day, and lost all that milk. It was definitely warm, so I had to throw it away.'

Christine's narrative displays the ongoing labour involved in managing, storing and properly handling peer-donated milk. She developed a routine to defrost milk twice each day to feed to her foster son Liam, taking care to make the best use of all the milk.

Recipients also established careful routines to prepare donor milk for feeding. Most defrosting and preparation practices were in accordance with ABM standards (Eglash et al 2017) and general breastmilk-handling guidelines (Reyes-Foster et al 2017). Rhonda described how she prepared peer-shared milk for her third child, Jaime, whom she fed only one bag of peer milk each day, to supplement his primary diet of infant formula:

> 'I just take one of the bags out and whatever's in that, I put it in and then I put the rest formula.... So, what I do is I take the milk out, the milk bag that I want to use for the next day, and I just put it, actually I'll take a couple of them out and put it in the refrigerator, so that they can defrost for 24 hours. And then I take that milk bag and I have a measuring cup, and I put it in the measuring cup in the sink and I run lukewarm water over it, so it kinda warms it up to room temperature for him. And then – 'cause I don't ever shake it or anything – and then I just swirl it around and put it in the bottle. And then I'll just add some formula to make an eight-ounce bottle. So that's how I prepare it. Lately the bags that I have usually have like three or four ounces in them. So, I just use one whole bag for a bottle and then I put the rest formula on top of it.... Sometimes I just run the water over it to make it room temperature or even maybe a little bit warmer, but I gradually warm it up. I don't put hot water on it or anything.'

Although only a few participants used peer milk to complement a mostly formula-based diet, Rhonda's narrative is nonetheless representative of the common preparation practices for defrosting and heating peer-shared milk. Like Rhonda, most recipients described some routine they followed for preparing the milk that was in accordance with ABM guidelines, which included defrosting the milk in the refrigerator or under warm water, heating it in water, and never putting it in a microwave.

Our respondents were familiar with ABM guidelines, although some confessed to knowingly deviating from them. Thelma, who is a CLC, explained the difference between what she tells clients is the 'right' thing to do and what she does in practice:

> 'You know, when moms ask, "When my baby doesn't finish the bottle, what should I do?" Well, the official answer is you should throw that milk away. Because one, it's been heated, and two, now your baby's germs from their mouth is inside of the bottle from the air going back and forth into the nipple, so you should throw it away. Me? What I do? I stick in the refrigerator and use it in the next feeding!'

The reality that sometimes life is too complicated and milk is too precious to do things perfectly was clear in our respondents' narratives. In some instances, the emotive value of shared milk superseded following guidelines to perfection.

Feeding

The final step in handling milk by recipients was feeding it to their babies. For some, as in Rhonda's story described earlier, feeding peer milk was a straightforward process. Rhonda's second baby, Susan, was bottle-fed a combination of formula and peer milk. Rhonda felt good about giving Susan some human milk as a supplement to formula to boost immunity and provide additional nutrition. Similarly, Christine, who fed peer milk to her foster baby Liam, also exclusively fed through a bottle. For these recipients and others in similar situations, the actual feeding of peer breastmilk was likely comparable to other bottle-feeding experiences, where mothers experimented with different types of bottles and observed their effects (Afflerback et al 2013), but did not feel particularly emotional about feeding their babies through a bottle.

However, for many recipients, feeding peer-shared milk was one component of a larger, more complex, feeding regimen. These complex feeding arrangements were typically among mothers who were trying to breastfeed, using peer breastmilk to supplement their own. A few utilized an SNS, a device designed to mimic the physical experience of breastfeeding between mother and child while the baby receives milk from a container through a tube attached at the mother's nipple. The goal of the SNS is for the mother and baby to gain the physical connection of breastfeeding, and for the baby to stimulate the mother's milk production by suckling on the breast, yet for the baby to be satiated with milk even if the mother's body does not produce enough.

Shirley was devastated when she discovered that she was not producing enough milk to sustain her second baby, Vivian. Having breastfeeding difficulties with her first, and eventually discovering peer milk sharing, she decided immediately that she would seek breastmilk again. Even after securing a continuous donor, Sara, Shirley still worked very hard to produce her own milk. During the course of the hour-and-a-half interview between Shirley and Shannon, Shirley fed Vivian using an SNS, then pumped the remaining milk that Vivian was unable to extract, and as the interview wrapped up she was preparing the SNS for another feeding. She explained the emotional toll of this extensive labour, as well as her rationale for feeding through the SNS:

> 'So, at some point, like around six weeks, I was like, "This pumping thing is not sustainable." I have an older son, we're going places, how am I supposed to maintain this pumping long term? What's the end game? And so I keep saying, "This is not sustainable." Yet here I am, she's gonna be four months old next week, and I'm still doing it. Because, when it comes down to it, I kind of don't know how to stop pumping. I know that sounds crazy, but I don't know how to stop. And so, I've continued this. We have a car adapter, so I'm driving down the road with my pumping bra on and the car adapter, or, you know, we're driving to some club meeting and I'm hooked up to the pump. We're going to the science centre and I'm like, "Come on, we've got to go to the nursing room." So, it's like, I've somehow sustained what I said was not sustainable. But every couple of weeks I have a breakdown about it and I'm like, "I have to give up, I have to. I need, somebody needs to tell me that it's okay to quit." And for some reason, every couple of weeks when I give myself permission to quit, then I'm like, "Okay I have permission to quit. I'm not going to quite yet, but I have permission to." So, at any moment I can. I know that sounds ridiculous, it's craziness, I mean it just is.'

Shirley's feeding routine was extensive, and it created ongoing emotional turmoil. She recognized the continuous time and energy – the labour – she dedicated to pumping and feeding as unsustainable yet had managed to sustain it for four months. She continued:

> 'So now I'm really only supplementing – and to be honest with you in the last several days I don't think I've supplemented with donor milk at all – which is unbelievable for me that I'm really almost at full supply. I mean, with tremendous effort, but I'm supplying her needs. For quite a while it was about three ounces of mine and one ounce of donor. Three ounces of mine, one ounce of donor. So, it was mostly mine, but I'm having to pump it all, she can't remove it. That's where we are. I exclusively pump. I mean, we use the SNS and I use a nipple shield so it's like, there is a lot of plastic involved in my breastfeeding experience, which just kills me. But, yeah, I'm using the nipple shield and the SNS, I'm basically pumping it out and then giving it back to her in the SNS. Because she will not just latch and just remove milk from me because of her oral issues and because of my flat nipple, and even with just the nipple shield, she still can't suck, she's still got some stuff going on.'

Shirley's description of her pumping and feeding routine highlights the vast effort she dedicates to breastfeeding, and the role of commercial technological devices – the breast pump, the SNS, and the nipple shield – that moderate her infant-feeding regimen. This use of consumer products and technological devices has become characteristic of breastfeeding in the 21st-century Global North (Boswell-Penc and Boyer 2007; Boyer 2010; Boyer and Boswell-Penc 2010; Stearns 2010; Afflerback et al 2013; Torres 2014; Lee 2018b).

When asked what the benefits are for her to use the SNS rather than feed her baby through a bottle, Shirley explained:

> 'Okay, several reasons. Number one because she has the oral issues that she has, I want her to get as much development in the muscle. I want her to have to work as hard as she can, you know, I want her to exercise every time she nurses. So, I want her at the breast. And it is emotionally easier on me to have my baby at the breast. So, the emotional cost to me of giving a bottle is pretty high. Whereas a lot of women wouldn't care, to me it is high. It was high for

> my son, but for him I tried the SNS. I didn't have great help with the SNS and nobody told me it's really hard at first and you have to really push through and figure it out, and so I gave up. I was so beyond overwhelmed and in the worst postpartum depression, like close to psychosis, horrible depression with him. It was too much. So, with him I had to just say, "I can't do the SNS," and I bottle-fed him. But again, the emotional cost was really high. We also, with him, I would nurse him first and then top off with the bottle. Now the thinking has kind of changed to be more, "Finish at the breast." I don't know if you are aware, now it's more like a recommendation of, "Feed first and finish at the breast" so that the breast remains a happy place. Because if the baby can't get, if the flow was slower through the breast, the baby gets angry and frustrated. And, so now the recommendation is, "Finish at the breast" so they're not as starving, they're happy to just comfort nurse longer. So that was my plan and with Vivian, number two came around and all this happened and you know, several people said, "Why don't you try the SNS?" I immediately went, "No, I'm not doing that. I'm not putting myself through that." But the emotional cost of giving the bottles and knowing that she was probably going to give up nursing, comfort nursing, sooner made me go, "Maybe I'll push through it and figure it out." And I'm so glad that I did.'

For Shirley, the physical and embodied labour involved in feeding Vivian through the SNS where she would be at the breast outweighed the emotional costs to her of feeding her through a bottle. Although this method took more work, especially in getting started and learning how to use the SNS, she was willing to exchange this labour for the emotional turmoil she felt over bottle feeding. Thelma also used an SNS, but she found her baby's latch issues prevented him from retrieving enough milk – "I had to squeeze the SNS into his mouth," she explained, and she ultimately started to bottle-feed him.

Digesting

Scholars who study breastfeeding as embodied practice (Schmied and Barclay 1999; Schmied and Lupton 2001; Shaw 2004b; Kelleher 2006; Hausman 2007; Stearns 2009, 2013; Ryan et al 2011; Lee 2018a, 2018b) suggest that the labour involved in breastfeeding depends not only on the mother's embodied work, but also the embodied work of the child who is being fed. In this conceptualization, the baby is as much an actor as the mother and the milk. We can see the baby as actor in the previous section on feeding, and their actions remain important as they interact with and become transformed by shared milk. They respond to what they are fed and communicate their reactions by grunting in pleasure as they eat, by crying and kicking when they have gas or feel unwell, by growing and gaining weight, or by failing to thrive. Parents learn to read these sometimes subtle cues and this in turn informs their feeding decisions.

It is often these cues that lead parents to seek donor milk in the first place. Mona Lisa didn't realize she wasn't producing enough milk until her baby, Ricardo, began showing symptoms of ill health. During a routine doctor's visit, the paediatrician found that Ricardo had lost 14% of his body weight and had high bilirubin levels, indicating jaundice. As a result, Ricardo had to return to the hospital. Mona Lisa was instructed to supplement her breastmilk with formula because of Ricardo's condition. She explained:

> 'I told my doula, "They're making me supplement him with formula. It's breaking my heart!" The first day I gave him formula, oh, his tummy was rumbling. I could tell he was just, I could tell he was not a happy camper. And he would strain like he was constipated. Oh! It was breaking my heart.'

By fussing, straining and indicating difficulties with digesting formula, Ricardo communicated cues that Mona Lisa read as unhappiness and physical discomfort. She associated this unhappiness and discomfort directly to the introduction of formula, and this led her to seek an alternative. Her doula referred her to Get Pumped for donor milk and she began her milk-sharing journey.

> 'I was able to get my first donor milk from Get Pumped and the first feeding I could tell it was a huge difference. He was happier. He was, you know, finally seemed content. He got his weight back up, thankfully. I was still supplementing him a little bit with formula 'cause I didn't get the milk until a little bit later but I could just tell. It was like night and day, the difference between the milk and the formula.'

Mona Lisa immediately saw that Ricardo was happier with human milk than he was with formula. As she began to feed him donor milk, she began to enter the milk sharing bio-communities of practice. Her pick-up spot for the Get Pumped donor milk happened to be the office of Dr Leila, who sees many pregnant and nursing patients. One day, when Mona Lisa was picking up milk, she met Raven. On another occasion, when Mona Lisa stopped by Dr Leila's office, Dr Leila had milk that had been donated directly to her, not Get Pumped, in her freezer, and offered it to Mona Lisa. Mona Lisa accepted and found that Ricardo seemed to respond very well to this milk.

> 'I fed him this milk and he just did so good. He did so good with it. I could tell he really liked this milk, because with some of the other milk that I'd had before he was like, spitting up a little bit. But this one in particular, I don't know what it was, I just could tell. So, I messaged Dr Leila, I said, "Hey, do you know the lady that dropped off that milk?" I'm like, "She doesn't have to give me her name or anything, but could I get an email so I can – I just want to send her an email just to thank her." She gave me Melanie's email address and I emailed her, saying, "Hey, I know you don't know me but I'm the one who actually ended up picking up your milk from Dr Leila's and I just can't thank you enough for your milk. My baby is doing great, he loved your milk!" And she emailed me back. She said, "This is the first time I've ever donated! I've been dumping all my supply. I'm glad because every time I dump the milk it, you know, it broke my heart. I dropped it off not knowing where it would go, you know I had no idea. I'm glad you got it." And I'm like, "Yeah, here's a picture of baby Ricardo, he's doing great." She's become pretty much my exclusive – my exclusive mommy.'

Something about Ricardo's reaction to Melanie's milk made Mona Lisa seek her out. She can't describe exactly what that reaction was, she simply says, "I just *knew*." Ricardo exhibited satisfaction and happiness in response to Melanie's milk, and Mona Lisa picked up on these feelings. She was able to establish a long-term milk sharing relationship with Melanie, who became Ricardo's exclusive donor.

By establishing an exclusive milk-sharing relationship with Melanie, Mona Lisa ended the other milk-sharing relationships she had developed. We observed a few other instances where recipients would not ask a particular donor for milk based on their intuitive feelings about the milk or their babies' responses to it. Elaine, one of the donors we interviewed, described such a scenario. Elaine had donated about 400 ounces to Sharon over the course of a few months, but then Sharon's baby Gabriel – who was receiving milk from multiple donors – started having digestive issues, so Sharon discontinued the milk-sharing relationship. Like Mona Lisa, Sharon may have developed an exclusive milk-sharing relationship, or she may have switched her baby to infant formula. Either way, she interpreted baby Gabriel's actions as cues about how he was responding to the milk and used this information to guide her decisions about what to feed him.

Another way in which babies communicate the effects of human milk to their parents is through their excretions as the milk travels through their bodies (Falls 2017; Marshall et al 2007; Stearns 2009). Most babies experience some degree of spit-up, so parents will monitor the frequency and amount to determine whether the milk is compatible with their babies. They observe and listen to their babies' bodies as their milk is digested, looking for discomfort and signs of gas or indigestion. Faeces produced by formula have a very different composition than those produced by human milk. Parents notice these changes in their babies' diapers and are motivated to continue receiving milk when the excretions match the descriptions provided by their medical providers, a process also noted by Falls (2017). In this way, recipient parents follow their babies' cues to guide their decisions on whether or not to continue active participation in milk sharing bio-communities of practice.

This chapter has traced milk from its production through to its digestion, illustrating along the way the myriad practices involved in peer milk sharing. We have considered the extensive embodied and emotional labour of both donors and recipients and, importantly, their babies. This labour is foundational to the emotional materiality of shared milk. In part, sharing milk is meaningful because it takes so much work to produce and procure. The extensive care donors and recipients take in producing, managing, transferring and feeding the milk speaks to its value, as both a material expression of emotion and human connection, and as a vital substance. The practices we present reflect the ways in which milk-sharing participants maintain milk-sharing bio-communities of practice. The interconnectedness and relationships of the bio-communities of practice are further explored in Chapter 5.

5

The Milk-Sharing Network

The Educated Mama, a closed Facebook group devoted to natural parenting and informed choice, is a busy place. With over 10,000 members, new posts devoted to questions of child development, baby sleep and cloth diapering appear constantly. Breastfeeding struggles are a frequent topic of conversation, and in these contexts milk sharing often comes up. In an age of visual storytelling and memes, one of the most visually striking posts observed are those of collages lovingly created by mothers whose babies have benefitted from donor milk. These visual stories present a narrative of interconnectedness, of babies connected to unrelated mothers and each other by the milk they consume. In this chapter, we explore the nature of these connections.

Foundational context

The first thing I (Beatriz) did when I found out I was pregnant with my oldest son was go on the internet. I spent hours reading up on pregnancy on websites like BabyCenter and The Bump. Before I was even out of my first trimester, I had devoted an inordinate amount of time to reading reviews for car seats, stroller, and bassinettes. I marvelled at the biological process of lactation and eagerly repeated to myself the mantra 'breast is best'. Home birth wasn't right for me, but when I saw that having a midwife-attended hospital birth reduced the chances of C-sections, I immediately decided that was the care I would seek – and then spent hours researching local nurse-midwives. Once I found a provider, I attended my appointments and read the pregnancy magazines in the lobby. I learned about attachment parenting – a style of parenting that encourages secure attachment through constant bonding and contact between baby and caretaker (Granju and Kennedy 1999; Sears and Sears 2001; Faircloth 2013) – and decided that was what I wanted to do. I saw people wearing their babies in little blue carriers and knew I wanted one too. As the months progressed, I was exposed to a series of discourses and objects that shaped my desires for the baby I was soon to have. Some of these ideas had to do with philosophies of child raising, but others were products I needed to purchase. Pregnancy was both about my changing identity as a mother but also as a consumer (Afflerback et al 2013, 2014; Han 2013; O'Donohoe et al 2013; Kehily and Martens 2014; Tiidenberg and Baym 2017).

Expectant parents navigate a complex set of often competing discourses that informs their decisions around all aspects of birth and infant care (Locke 2009, 2018; Malacrida and Boulton 2012; Porter et al 2012; Hausman 2014; Foss 2017). Alongside 'intensive mothering', 'natural' and 'biomedical' perspectives fuel the discursive marketplace from which caretakers draw their information. Once they know they are expecting, many parents spend hours reading and interacting with an array of literature, websites and social networks. Facebook groups form around particular due dates, and parents may soon find themselves building connections and interacting through social media with other expectant parents who share various interests (Johnson 2014; Asiodu et al 2015; Lupton et al 2016; Locatelli 2017; Thomas et al 2018; Eagle 2019). These common interests often revolve around mode of birth – out-of-hospital versus in-hospital, vaginal versus C-section – or infant-feeding plans –formula, exclusive breastmilk, or a little of both – or just general ideas about lifestyle – baby wearing versus strollers, cry-it-out versus bed sharing, cloth diapers versus disposable. Breastmilk sharing exists in this milieu of discourse and practice, as parents navigate this marketplace of ideas and choose the decisions that best resonate with their own values and experiences. Alongside discourses found online and in literature, parents receive unsolicited magazines, formula samples and other kinds of literature at home and at their healthcare providers' offices.

These physical, virtual and discursive realms form the foundational context from which milk sharing emerges. Some aspects of this context could be argued are universal, at least in the Global North, where websites, social media posts, parenting books and magazines, and dominant parenting 'theories' tend to be consistent with intensive mothering (Hays 1996) in various ways (Song et al 2012; Faircloth 2013; Johnson 2014; Pedersen 2016; Carter 2017; Hookway et al 2017; Tiidenberg and Baym 2017; Eagle 2019). Other aspects of this context are more specific to country or region, with variations based on healthcare systems, types of providers, and prevalence of breastfeeding or other infant-feeding practices. In the US, the context is also determined by privilege, as the ability to pay for a doula, enroll in hypnobirthing classes, or select the medical provider of one's choice varies by race, ethnicity, socioeconomic status and region. Within the broader US context, Florida is distinct in that out-of-hospital birth is readily available and covered by both private insurance and Medicaid. In practice, this means that almost all women with low-risk pregnancies, regardless of income, have the option to pursue birth at home or in a birth centre with a midwife.[1] In Florida, nearly 2% of babies are born at home or in a birthing centre (MacDorman and Declerq 2019). Although our research sample had an overrepresentation of parents who opted for out-of-hospital birth, the majority of our research participants (70%) planned to and gave birth in hospitals. Anyone who has been a patient in both an out-of-hospital midwifery and an obstetric practice will notice that the adjacent discourses – the posters on the walls, the types of magazines and other literature available, the types of providers to which patients are referred – are quite different from one another. Whereas an obstetric practice will expose patients to biomedically oriented discourses and products like pharmaceuticals, a midwifery practice is more likely to offer products and services from other 'natural-living' practitioners and companies (Macdonald 2006; Simonds et al 2007). For those who can afford it, birth doulas and lactations consultants can also prove to be a crucial link to other, lesser known resources (Waggoner 2011; Torres 2015).

Thus, the foundational context contains within it both the 'mainstream' as well as 'natural' birthing and parenting discourses, products and communities. Here, based on their own interests, expectant parents encounter seemingly endless possibilities. Most encounter a clear message that 'breast is best', as breastfeeding promotion has been taken up more or less unanimously by maternity care providers, pregnancy and parenting guides, health organizations, and state and local governments (Wall 2001; Kukla 2006; Wolf 2007, 2010; Crossley 2009; Jansson 2009; Knaak 2010; Waggoner 2011; Carter 2017). However, the consistency of messaging and its implementation in healthcare practices that support breastfeeding vary widely. Many women are told they *should* breastfeed but are not provided with the education or support on how to do it (Kelleher 2006; Lee 2007, 2008; Marshall et al 2007; Cross-Barnet et al 2012; Stearns 2013). Many receive contradictory messaging through the aggressive marketing of infant formula, sometimes given to them as a 'gift' from healthcare providers, and many hospitals still engage in practices that undermine breastfeeding, such as unnecessary separation of mother and baby, introducing pacifiers, or supplementing with formula (Brady 2012; Cross-Barnet et al 2012; Hausman 2014; Ryan et al 2017).

Thus, some institutions inadvertently promote formula feeding, or undermine women's efforts to breastfeed, even while giving the overt message that 'breast is best'.

Within this foundational context, the presence of HMBANA milk banks sets the stage for peer milk sharing by establishing an institutionally and medically endorsed option for feeding infants an unrelated stranger's milk. Although there are many distinctions between the two practices, and many who promote milk banking disavow peer milk sharing, the presence of milk banks nevertheless hints that another human's milk might be a healthier food for infants than artificial formula.

Perhaps not immediately apparent to new expectant parents, but also very present in this foundation, is peer milk sharing. Among the endless groups, networks, organizations and products available are the milk-sharing networks Human Milk 4 Human Babies and Eats on Feets (Akre et al 2011; Cassidy 2012a). The human milk marketplace Only The Breast and its darker underbelly, Craigslist, also exist in the foundational context. Locally, Get Pumped and the Mothers' Milk Bank of Florida are visible in the community – both organizations host charity and community events, and their flyers, directed at potential donors, can be found in the offices of local obstetricians, midwives and alternative care providers. Both of these local organizations also maintain active Facebook pages.

While cloth diapering, baby wearing and breastfeeding are very visible in the discursive realm, milk sharing is not a readily visible practice. As Chapter 3 described, many caregivers do not discover milk sharing until they begin to struggle with breastfeeding or when they find themselves overwhelmed with milk. However, they do belong to wider networks where interactions involving milk sharing take place. Social media has become one of the most powerful devices by which people not only research particular topics but discover broader global networks with which they choose to connect (Lupton et al 2016; Fuchs 2017). Groups such as Dairy Queens and The Leaky Boob, alongside pages like Black Women do Breastfeed and Natural Parenting, feature the creation and exchange of memes, personal testimonies and media reports that shape this discourse. Particular times of year, such as World Breastfeeding Week, Black Breastfeeding Week and World Milk Sharing Week, elicit increased activity and communication. These engagements are not one-directional: caregivers who belong to these networks also participate in them by creating and sharing content or by engaging with shared content and each other (Locatelli 2017). A mother may share her story of struggle on the breastfeeding support group Dairy Queens and among the advice she receives is a suggestion of milk sharing. Others might disagree, and a lively conversation about the topic may ensue. Another mother 'lurking' may be reading the exchanges without participating, and this may be the first time she ever hears of milk sharing. Like some of our participants, she might file the thought away in the back of her mind, "just in case". This discursive realm is accessible to nearly anyone with access to a computer or a cell phone. And while the demographics of social media are changing – younger people tend to participate in the image-heavy Instagram or the ephemeral Snapchat (Perrin and Anderson 2019) – Facebook continues to provide a virtual platform to 2.45 billion users around the world (Statista 2020). However, even as the average age of new mothers is rising, mothers of babies are in an age group that tends to use multiple social media platforms. In addition to the extensive use of Facebook to facilitate milk sharing that we outline in this book, new mothers use other social media forums to gain and share information about parenting. For example, the #breastfeeding hashtag reflects over 3.9 million posts on Instagram. The Spanish-language hashtags #lactancia and #amamantar have 466,000 and 76,400 posts respectively, and the Portuguese #aleitamentomaterno has 246,000. These media platforms are an important part of contemporary social life.

As a major metropolitan area, Orlando has a lot to offer expectant parents –major hospitals, thriving midwifery communities, and several birth centres. Besides the major chains, parents are able to obtain natural and fair-trade goods from a variety of local small businesses and large corporations. Indoor play areas and many, many parks abound. The city also hosts a children's science museum, the Orlando Science Center, and a variety of other family-friendly spaces. Finally, the theme parks, especially Disney, are an important part of the area's cultural and economic life. The cultural milieu surrounding expectant parents is rich, diverse and full of possibilities for chance encounters.

Milk-sharing emerges

I was 14 weeks' pregnant with Rowan the first time Shannon and I met over coffee at the University of Central Florida campus café to talk about collaborating on a new project. When we realized the potential of studying milk sharing, we both recognized the opportunity presented by the fact that I would soon have a nursling of my own: I could combine mothering my newborn with our research by attending breastfeeding support groups once he was born. This would facilitate my access to some of the communities Shannon was already involved in, and potentially open new doors to communities closer to my house and newer cohorts of breastfeeding and milk-sharing parents. At the time, I did not know I was going to once again experience difficulties breastfeeding, but I intended to visit these groups regardless because I had found them to be a valuable social outlet when my first son, Aydin, was an infant. When Rowan was six weeks old and I finally felt well enough to drive – and when it was already apparent that my supply would not be able to keep up with his demand – I decided to attend my first breastfeeding support group as both a mother and a researcher: participant observation at its finest. I arrived at Holistic Health midwifery practice shortly before the Lactating Mamas group was about to begin. Back in 2014, Holistic Health had not yet opened its second birth centre in downtown Orlando. The practice had a midwifery office used for prenatal visits and well-woman care outside the city, and a beautiful birth centre in a renovated craftsman-style house closer to the beach. Lactating Mamas met twice a week, once at each location. On this particular day, I attended the breastfeeding support meeting at the midwifery office. Although this was the first time I met Shonda, her reputation preceded her: her Lactating Mamas Facebook group was an active, lively space, and the doulas and midwives I had come to know over the course of my second pregnancy and childbirth all spoke highly of her commitment to helping all women breastfeed. Shonda is one of the few Black IBCLC's active in the area. She is committed to reproductive justice and often speaks about the importance of supporting breastfeeding for Black women. Importantly, at the time that she had a busy practice as an IBCLC, she was also employed as a lactation consultant by a local county Health Department, to support breastfeeding among WIC programme recipients.

The Holistic Health midwifery practice was located at one end of historic town's main street, in a one-storey 1970s office complex with floor-to-ceiling windows overlooking the lake. The meeting took place in a quiet alcove off the main waiting area. Children's toys sat neatly in a corner next to the couches, and some of the mothers with newborns who came carting toddlers made quick use of them. On this late March morning, I and five other women were in attendance. One of the first things I noticed was that Shonda and I were the only women of colour in the group –all of the other mothers were white. The meeting started, as many breastfeeding support group meetings do, with a brief introduction by the meeting leader. Each of us took turns, introducing ourselves, our babies, and our breastfeeding experiences. When my turn came, I described my recent struggles to produce enough milk for Rowan and explained that I had had to begin supplementing with formula. Some of the mothers who attended that day were not struggling at the time but had struggled previously and had received support from Shonda and the group. Others were struggling with oversupply or had babies with a tongue-tie or a weak suck.

It was very clear that Shonda was in charge. As each one of us spoke, Shonda offered her expert feedback and advice. For instance, when I spoke, she offered to assess Rowan's latch to make sure he was latching properly, and then said we could talk about milk supply after everyone had introduced themselves. The last mother who spoke was a young blond woman in her 20s. Her baby boy was about three months old, and she explained that, like me, she was not producing enough milk to exclusively feed him. She nursed him as she spoke, and when he started fussing she pulled out a small cooler from her bag. "It has been hard," she explained as she pulled a bag of milk out of the cooler, "but thankfully, my friend here has been able to donate. So, he is getting a few ounces of donor milk after every feed." She gestured to the woman sitting next to her. I soon learned that the two had met at Lactating Mamas and that the donor would bring milk to the meeting. I then realized that she, too, had brought a cooler with her. Shonda nodded in affirmation as this mother spoke. When she was done, she spoke about the struggle to exclusively breastfeed, and acknowledged milk sharing as an option that was available to mothers who could not produce enough milk.

Although I purported to attend this meeting as both a researcher and a mother, the truth is that it is actually rather difficult to combine these tasks. I had to deal with my own difficulties, and at that time I had not decided to start using donor milk. In my own struggle, I did not attempt to speak with this donor–recipient dyad, and so I know very little about their story. What I do know is that this was the first time I had attended a breastfeeding support group, and that milk sharing was not only discussed, but happened right in front of me. I later learned that Holistic Health keeps a freezer full of donated milk. The office serves as a drop-off and pick-up point for Get Pumped, and the midwives solicit milk from screened donors for mothers of infants in need of milk. They allow screened donors like Sara to drop off whatever surplus they have for mothers who may need it. In our own life experiences, Shannon and I both found milk sharing taking place in plain sight in breastfeeding support groups at different birth centres. When I attended Lactating Mamas, it was clear that Shonda had not actively participated in facilitating the exchange, but her tacit approval from her expert position legitimated and normalized the practice for those of us in attendance. During our research we interviewed Madeline, a midwife and owner of the birth centre, who made clear that most of the milk sharing was facilitated through the midwives themselves, not through the Lactating Mamas group, or through Shonda.

For health professionals like Shonda, milk sharing presents a challenge. In her personal life, she first became involved in milk sharing when she nursed her sister's baby. However, in accordance with IBCLC professional guidelines, Shonda is not supposed to promote peer milk sharing, although she can support informed choice. She navigated this challenge carefully, even in the way she spoke about milk sharing in our interview:

> 'In my profession as an IBCLC, I don't support non-formal milk sharing. I cannot support it, so I always direct [my clients] to a milk bank.... I educate my clients on that. Now, if they decide to go another route, that is on them.... I do have the Lactating Mamas support group, and sometimes they post there asking for milk, but that is of their will, it doesn't come from me. If they happen to connect in the group, that is on them.'

Thus, although she does not directly support milk sharing outside of the context of milk banks, Shonda facilitates a space where milk sharing frequently takes place. Her Lactating Mamas Facebook group has over 800 members, and the group meets face to face every week.

Shonda is not the only IBCLC in town who is aware of and at least tacitly supports milk sharing. River, who is white, is also an IBCLC with a busy private and hospital-based practice. She initially learned about milk sharing after giving birth to her youngest daughter, when another mother in her circle suffered an aneurism and was unable to continue nursing her baby. In response to a request for donor milk, River donated her own milk to that baby. She eventually became involved with Get Pumped and served on the organization's board for a number of years. She explained that in her professional practice she often encounters people who have an excess of milk, and also people who need it:

> 'Just the other day I had a client that told me she had about 250 ounces and she didn't want to go through the process of becoming a milk donor for a milk bank so she asked if I had anybody that I knew of who needed milk. So, I connected

> her with one of my other clients that needed it and, you know, the rest is history.'

Based on her interview, it is clear that River supports milk sharing overtly, not just tacitly. By the same token, River's involvement with Get Pumped and her role in the organization's activities and policies highlight the ways in which lactation professionals such as River and Shonda can play an important role in promoting and educating women on best practices for safety in milk sharing. Several of the donors and recipients in our study were also lactation counsellors. However, these are not the only professionals with proximity to milk sharing. River also noted that doulas frequently play a key role in making milk-sharing connections, and that even some medical providers, such as a local paediatrician known for supporting 'naturally minded' parenting decisions, are supportive of parents who resort to donor milk. In my own experience, my first paediatrician in Orlando, who was part of a naturally minded practice, was also supportive of our choice to use donor milk and it was my doula who first suggested I consider donor milk for my baby. Shannon's paediatrician, who maintains a busy practice on the other side of town, encourages all patients of newborns to have a consultation with River, whose practice is housed in his office, and was mentioned in several interviews with donors and recipients as knowing and supporting his patients' participation in peer milk sharing. Emerging research suggests that these practices are not unique to Central Florida, but that many maternity care providers, lactation consultants and paediatricians throughout the Global North tacitly facilitate milk sharing (Shaw and Morgan 2017; Cassar-Uhl and Liberatos 2018; O'Sullivan et al 2018; Perrin et al 2018; Palmquist et al 2019).

Our participants also reported encountering milk sharing in a variety of different places, some more unexpected than others. For instance, a local hospital hosts a weekly breastfeeding luncheon, and a group of regular attendees created a Facebook group named after the luncheon event. Because breastfeeding is a largely accepted practice, with nearly 82.6% of mothers reporting ever breastfeeding (CDC 2018), this event attracts all kinds of caregivers who want to breastfeed, not an exclusively naturally minded cohort. Nevertheless, Isabella and Elaine both encountered milk sharing in either the face-to-face or the Facebook group. Naturally minded parents have many opportunities to overlap with one another, and are often provided services by a small network of providers who all tend to know one another, such as people like Shonda, River and Dr Leila. Dr Leila's office – which, interestingly enough, now occupies Holistic Health midwifery's former space in the office complex overlooking the lake – is in a halfway point between the Orlando metropolitan area and Florida's east coast communities. The town is also home to the well-known Mother's Love Birth Center. Like Holistic Health, Mother's Love is also known to collect milk and distribute it to their clients who need it. Mother's Love also hosts a regular breastfeeding support group, Breast Friends, which holds weekly in-person meetings, and has a private Facebook group with about 400 members.

Thus, the lines between local online and face-to-face networks can be blurred. Many conversations start online and move into the 'real world', and vice versa. And these conversations aren't only happening in breastfeeding support groups such as the ones described earlier. For instance, ICAN hosts a weekly support meeting for mothers who have experienced C-sections. While this group is not a breastfeeding support group, breastfeeding support does occur as part of its meetings – Rhonda was first introduced to milk sharing because she saw it taking place at an ICAN meeting. The private Facebook group Volusia Moms Network hosts regular in-person meet-ups, and The Breastfeeding Project, an organization both Beatriz and Shannon were involved with, hosts monthly social gatherings. In addition, other large-scale events, such as the Big Latch On and the Great Cloth Diaper Change, bring similarly minded people in direct contact with one another. For our participants, milk sharing appeared in many online and offline spaces, including natural parenting Facebook groups, breastfeeding support groups connected to the Mother's Love Birth Center, Holistic Health, and the non-profit organization Get Pumped, as well as through Dr Leila's practice. Like an open secret, milk sharing is easy to come by if one knows where to look.

While our sample tended to be skewed towards white and relatively affluent mothers, we encountered several instances where milk sharing was discussed in other contexts. In 2014, Shonda, who was working at the Health Department in the WIC programme, invited us to set up a table on behalf of The Breastfeeding Project. The mission of The Breastfeeding Project was to provide an alternative to the marketing bags full of formula most new mothers received in hospitals and paediatrician's offices. To this end, we created bags full of breastfeeding resources, including information about support groups, local providers and breastfeeding educational materials. The bags also contained a water bottle and other 'goodies' to support breastfeeding such as lanolin and a rice compress. They were distributed by breastfeeding-friendly healthcare providers to new and expectant mothers, or by The

Breastfeeding Project volunteers at events targeting new and expectant mothers. For World Breastfeeding Week, Shonda invited us to the local Health Department to set up a table and distribute our bags to the WIC lactation counsellors who travelled from all over the state to attend an educational workshop.

With Beatriz's baby in his wrap, we eagerly set up our table and began to distribute our bags. We also distributed a flyer containing a link to the online survey we were conducting on milk sharing. As we handed it out, several of the WIC counsellors stopped to chat with us. "Oh, milk sharing!," exclaimed one of the counsellors, "we really want to support it, but we aren't allowed to." Another counsellor chuckled, "That's right, so as soon as it comes up in group I tell them, 'You can't talk about it in here, but if you want to take it outside and discuss it, I can't stop you!'"

We soon realized that although WIC counsellors are not allowed to support or facilitate peer milk sharing, at least some of those we came into contact with tacitly supported the practice. Again, the nature of milk sharing as an open secret – something that many do but few talk about – became clear, as did its presence in the foundational context, not hidden but not obvious: emergent and connected through practice.

Connected through practice

Within the foundational context described earlier, caregivers who give and receive milk, and the children they feed, together form milk sharing bio-communities of practice. They are communities of practice because they develop around a common goal of feeding human milk to babies and children, and they are bio-communities of practice because they achieve their goals by sharing human biological material. Donors who give milk and recipient children who consume it are connected through milk, establishing a bio-intimate connection as the donors' biological material enters the child's body and transforms it (Shaw 2019; Shaw and Morgan 2017). Individuals who participate in the practice of milk sharing but who do not share milk with each other are connected through the practice, establishing a collective biosociality that exists at both the local and global levels (Cassidy 2012a; Shaw and Morgan 2017, Shaw 2017, 2019).

Local bio-communities of practice

In the milk-sharing bio-communities we observed, milk sharing took place mostly at the level of the local community. Even people who initially connected with each other online, with only a few exceptions, eventually met in person to transfer milk. It was also within the local community where many participants learned about milk sharing, and where milk sharing emerged as an acceptable alternative to feeding formula or discarding excess breastmilk. This learning, and the subsequent sharing of milk that took place, often emerged from the local foundational context of interconnected maternity care and alternative healthcare providers, and breastfeeding support and other parenting and natural parenting groups, supported by both their online and offline presence. From this foundational context, individuals learned about and participated in peer milk sharing, thereby joining, and sometimes forming their own, local milk-sharing bio-communities of practice.

The healthcare providers who served as central facilitators recruited many participants into milk-sharing bio-communities, fostering not just the exchange of milk, but also the creation and maintenance of community. Many participants learned about milk sharing from these providers, who educated their patients about milk sharing and helped connect them to the people and spaces where milk sharing takes place. Several participants learned about milk sharing from Dr Leila, a local chiropractor and breastfeeding advocate who is well known within the birth community for her chiropractic work with pregnant women, babies and children. She hosts monthly breastfeeding support groups and other educational events, sometimes with a guest speaker, focused on a specific topic and manages a local Facebook group focused on natural health and holistic remedies. Dr Leila has a regular, home-size refrigerator in her office, where she stores her lunch, water and other items for personal use. She donates some of her freezer space to Get Pumped, providing a convenient location for donors and recipients who live northeast of Orlando or closer to the beach to drop off and pick up milk, and she facilitates direct milk exchanges between donors and recipients. She is an advocate of human breastmilk feeding, connecting her clients with healthcare services that support breastfeeding, such as lactation consultants or paediatricians who are known for correcting tongue-tie or lip-tie, and recruiting donors for Get Pumped or connecting them directly to people she knows who need milk.

Ashley, who was introduced to milk sharing through Dr Leila, and donated milk to four recipients, described how she experienced the local milk-sharing bio-communities of practice:

> 'I really learned about milk sharing through Dr Leila. I mean, I knew about it before, but I didn't realize how many people were actually requesting and using milk from

> other moms. So, I'd say I learned mostly through Leila. And then I joined some of the groups where moms share milk and just to see this whole community of people helping each other, it was definitely different than what I thought of. And even though everyone is local, it's usually on Facebook that I see it, and where I connect with people. The one time it was through Leila there was a mom who needed milk who she connected me with. Another time it was through the Lactating Mamas Facebook group, that somebody had posted there. I think that might have been where I posted that I was going to give milk and that's how I met the one mom in Orlando who I gave milk to, who needed it. So that time I posted that I had extra milk and then somebody posted someone else's name, and then that was how I ended up getting in touch with her to give her the milk. That Facebook group is a private, closed group, not like Human Milk 4 Human Babies or Eats on Feets where anyone can go in and see what people are posting. It's a closed group that you have to be accepted into in order to view the posts or participate. And really, I mean, a lot of those moms are also on a couple other groups, like Breast Friends support group and all the other ones. But on those groups you kind of know people in the group in a way, because it's all closed groups, none of them are open. And in these groups, you see the same people over and over. So, it's kind of like a community of women that are in these different groups. So, the one mom, the one I met through Lactating Mamas who I donated to in Orlando, she was new to the group because her baby was just a newborn at the time. So, I hadn't seen her in the groups before, but now I'm seeing her on all these other pages as well.'

By introducing Ashley to milk sharing, and the Facebook groups where it is facilitated, Dr Leila connected her with a whole community of people engaging in similar sets of practices. Although the groups are not designed to facilitate milk sharing, but instead focus on breastfeeding and other aspects of parenting, they provide a space for those who participate in milk sharing to connect with one another. Ashley was surprised by the community aspect of milk sharing that she observed online, particularly that so many people were working together to help each other. Although most of the people were unknown to her beforehand, she started seeing the same people over and over, posting in different groups, and they became familiar over time. This sense of familiarity, along with a shared orientation toward parenting and a collaborative orientation toward meeting those goals, fostered a sense of community (Cassidy and El Tom 2010; Cassidy 2012a; Falls 2017; Shaw and Morgan 2017; Shaw 2019). In this way, milk-sharing participants were connected through practice: they did not all share milk directly with one another, but they engaged in similar practices that were motivated by shared goals.

Mona Lisa, whom I (Shannon) met at a coffee shop on the southwest side of Orlando, was connected to a different group of healthcare professionals who introduced her to milk sharing. These professionals knew Dr Leila, and they collaborated at larger community events and online, but they mainly provided services to women in the Orlando metropolitan area. Mona Lisa described how she was introduced to the milk-sharing community in Central Florida when her baby was only a few days old:

> 'Once the test results came back, the doctor told me I needed to supplement with formula to get his weight back up and that I needed to go get him treated for jaundice. So, at that point I wasn't sleeping, I was crying, I was very emotional, and I just had no idea what I was doing. And thankfully, my doula was the one that brought it up. I was very close to her, and she helped me so much postpartum. But luckily, the community is so big here in Central Florida, but I had no clue until I got into it and I decided on a home birth and I got myself a midwife and a doula. And there were several doulas that ended up helping me afterwards, I had Abigail help me, Mariana, Gina, Connie, all of them.'

As the conversation progressed, Mona Lisa and I figured out that we knew many of the same doulas and midwives, and that I had interviewed her first donor. She summarized, "That just shows how small the community is, right? Like it's big and thriving, but it's small at the same time." As we became more enmeshed in the natural childbirth community in the area, we soon identified the ways in which birth professionals – doulas, midwives, chiropractors and lactation consultants – were connected with one another. One of the ways was geographic – people such as Dr Leila, who is located in a relatively central point and knows birth professionals in both Orlando and the

Florida coast, for instance. Another was linguistic: Mariana, a lactation consultant, and Claudia, a midwife, were both native Spanish speakers. Although both were located in the central part of Orlando and had both an English- and Spanish-speaking client base, they were also connected to the large Spanish-speaking community in Kissimmee, where a Spanish-language ICAN chapter regularly meets and its leader, Andrea, is also a birth doula attending VBACs in the area. During the course of our research, we became aware of the presence of these other communities, but unfortunately were unable to learn more about them for this project. However, these multiple, interconnected and co-present communities of practice exist in the foundational context of milk sharing and are other possible sites of emergence.

For Mona Lisa, the connectedness of community was an important part of milk sharing. She continued, describing her experiences with the community aspects of milk sharing, and discussing the motivations behind the practice:

> 'I just think that, I don't know how to explain it, but the intention of milk sharing is so kind. When it comes down to why people are doing this, why women are doing this, and to get down to the source and the reason of why we're doing it and why women are donating milk and receiving it, you'll realize the intentions are kind and pure and out of just sheer community and sisterhood. That's what I've gotten from all the women that I've met and that's why I've yet to hear someone buying milk over the internet so blindly as I see in the news because you have to be very desperate or be living somewhere so remote that you don't have that community of women. And again, just talking off of my own experience, that's the best thing of all, especially being a single mom, that all these women just reached out to me and shared milk with me. And just to have that connection really helped me get through this. And with Tamara, who donates milk to me regularly, I can't thank her enough. We've really become friends out of it, and I take her out to dinner, and I give her gift cards and other stuff to show her how grateful I am.'

Mona Lisa highlights that the motivations for participating in milk-sharing bio-communities of practice is not just to feed children breastmilk, but to help mothers, parents and other caregivers within the community. The interpersonal connections and sense of community bonding is not simply a by-product of milk sharing, but is a central motivating characteristic that drives participation, not only in the communities we studied, but in milk-sharing communities across the Global North (Cassidy 2012a, 2012b; Thorley 2012; Palmquist 2015; Falls 2017; Shaw and Morgan 2017; Gribble 2018; Wilson 2018; Shaw 2019).

Consistent with the communities of practice model, some of those who become participants in the communities recruit new members, educating them about the practices and encouraging their participation. Mona Lisa described an instance where she recruited someone to become a donor.

> 'I'm very good friends with Sherrie, one of the girls that works at my leasing office at my apartment complex. We were talking one day, and she didn't know that I was getting donor milk and it was at a point that I was running low. She was telling me, "I feel bad for my very good [friend] Bree. She pumps so much milk, she doesn't know what to do with it." She goes, "Poor thing carries pumps in her car, she has pumps everywhere, milk everywhere, and she doesn't know what to do with it." I'm like, "Is your friend healthy?" [We both laugh.] "How much dairy does she eat?" And she's looking at me so weird, and I'm like, "I don't know if you know about this, but there's a huge community where you can donate that milk. There's a lot of mommies that would appreciate that, one of them being me." So, then she put me in contact with Bree, and she became my next donor.'

Milk-sharing participants recruited new members to the communities they identified as having extra milk or whom they observed struggling with breastfeeding. As shown in Chapter 3, exposure and recruitment can take place online or in face-to-face settings. In practice, this means that members of milk-sharing bio-communities of practice are connected by their practice at both local and global scales. In this sense, the bio-communities of practice are similar to imagined communities in which members feel they are part of something larger than their immediate surroundings or communities (Cassidy and El Tom 2010; Shaw and Morgan 2017; Shaw 2019). Thanks to online social networks, these imagined communities are made real through online communication and engagement.

Global bio-communities of practice

Milk-sharing bio-communities of practice that form on a local level where milk is shared converge on a global level (Cassidy 2012a). People across the world who participate in the practice of milk sharing make up a global collective of milk-sharing bio-communities of practice. Connected by practice, they engage in a common set of activities motivated by a commitment to breastmilk feeding and a collective desire to work together to achieve breastmilk-feeding goals.

The global connectedness of people who share milk is not an unintended by-product of human milk sharing at the local level: it was an integral part of the vision of internet-based milk sharing organizations (Cassidy 2012a). Human Milk 4 Human Babies is designed to be a global network that facilitates breastmilk sharing at the local level through geographically based webpages, encouraging participants to 'think globally, share locally', yet the organizations themselves reflect the mantra of 'thinking locally and acting globally' (Cassidy 2012a: 236, 238). Similarly, the website for Eats on Feets states: 'By maintaining a global network, supporting families, reaching out to local communities, policy makers, professionals and again, people like YOU, it is our goal that community based breastmilk sharing continues to grow and be recognized as a normal and vital part of human life.'

People across the world who are connected by practice reiterate their membership in global milk-sharing bio-communities by subscribing to global networks, sharing memes and news articles related to milk sharing, and posting images that represent their own milk-sharing practices on social media. By sharing information about their own milk sharing, they educate others in their extended social networks about milk sharing, including the practices themselves and the underlying values that drive it. They disseminate this information to others, who at some point might find themselves needing milk or having excess to give or knowing someone who does. By spreading information, participants contribute to the perpetuation of milk-sharing bio-communities of practice.

Some participants described a sense of connectedness they felt with others at both the local and the global levels based on their mutual participation in peer milk sharing. Samantha researched milk sharing while she was pregnant with her third child after her first two had jaundice during their first few days after birth. She eventually established a healthy milk supply, but had difficulty producing colostrum, and as a result, her first two children were supplemented with formula in hospital to help fight their jaundice. To avoid having to feed formula to her third child, Franklin, Samantha posted a request for colostrum on the local Human Milk 4 Human Babies Facebook page. Within 48 hours, Kirsten, who had given birth at home the week before, responded to her request. The two met in the parking lot of Babies 'R Us, and Kirsten gave Samantha eight ounces of colostrum. Samantha was grateful for this gift, as it allowed her to avoid feeding Franklin formula, and she became a milk donor to a recipient she met through Human Milk 4 Human Babies once her milk supply was established. She explained her sense of connectedness to others who share milk:

> 'I feel like I've kind of joined that tribe whenever I started looking into Human Milk 4 Human Babies and Eats on Feets. And then one of my friends in the baby-wearing group that I'm a part of, Heidi, posted that she had received donor milk because she had IGT.[2] And I was like, "Oh really?" So, we got to talking about our experiences with milk sharing and I feel like it kind of gives you something to talk about, something to bond over on a certain level. So, we all kind of, it gives you a little tribe, I guess. We all feel like we have a common goal that we're working towards, to feed babies as much breastmilk as we can.'

Samantha felt she had joined the milk-sharing "tribe" when she started perusing the public Facebook pages of milk-sharing organizations. She learned about how milk sharing took place by reading the recommended guidelines on the organizations' official websites and observing interactions on the Facebook pages. By entering the world of milk sharing, Samantha felt that she had found a group with whom she belonged. Connected by practice, she shared a common goal with others across the state and across the world who share milk to provide as much human milk as possible to babies, and to do so in a collective way. This biosociality also fostered relationships at the local level, where Samantha felt a special bond with Heidi based on their mutual participation in milk sharing.

Connected through milk

Whereas all caregivers and children throughout the world who engage in peer milk sharing are connected through practice, those who engage directly with each other are connected through milk. As milk travels from a donor's body to a recipient baby, it not only transforms the baby's body as a vital substance, but it connects people on social and ontological levels (Falls 2017; Shaw 2017, 2019; Shaw and Morgan 2017). This view of breastmilk as a vessel of human relationships and connectivity transcends contemporary Euroamerican logic. Across societies and throughout human history, it is commonly a close relative who breastfeeds an infant when a mother's milk is not available, and kinship bonds are often formed through the sharing of milk among non-relatives (Lozoff 1983; Parkes 2001; Long 2003; Shaikh and Ahmed 2006; Cassidy and El Tom 2010; Ramli and Ibrahim 2010; Gribble 2013, 2018; Hewlett and Winn 2014; Thorley 2014; Onat and Karakoc 2019). Cultural norms that define close relatives but not strangers as figures whose milk can appropriately substitute a mother's own speak to a shared understanding – one that transcends time and place – of human milk as an element of kin making and connection (Falls 2017; Shaw 2017, 2019; Shaw and Morgan 2017; Gribble 2018; Wilson 2018). Donors throughout our study described a unique connection with recipient parents and the children who consumed their milk, and recipients likewise felt a sense of connectedness with the donors whose milk their children consumed. Within these relationships, individuals are connected through milk.

Bio-intimacy

The donating mother and recipient child dyad makes up the smallest and most bio-intimate unit within milk-sharing bio-communities of practice. Milk flows from the body of the donor to the body of the recipient baby, transforming the baby's physicality, and establishing a bio-intimate connection between the two. However, the biological material itself is not a vector of human social relationships. Instead, the meanings associated with bio-intimacy are shaped by broader societal definitions of breastmilk, family and friendship, which are negotiated in the contexts where milk sharing unfolds (Shaw and Morgan 2017; Shaw 2019). In several other contexts where biological and reproductive materials are transferred, such as egg and sperm donation, gestational surrogacy, live kidney donation and breastmilk banking, the meanings of the transfer and the resulting social relationships between donors and recipients are shaped by institutional and sometimes legal guidelines (Carroll 2014; Harrison 2016; Kroløkke and Peterson 2017; Shaw 2019). Without institutional regulatory guidelines in the context of peer milk sharing, donors and recipient caregivers negotiate these meanings themselves. The relationships created through bio-intimate connections are widely variable, and they are moderated by recipient caregivers, who develop their own relationships and varying sense of connectedness with donors.

The bio-intimate connections between donor and recipient child can be seen in the effects the milk has on the child (Falls 2017; Shaw and Morgan 2017; Shaw 2019). These effects are typically first observed by the recipient caregiver as the donor's milk changes the recipient child's body. As described in the preceding chapters, recipient parents in our study reported seeing the transformative effects of donated breastmilk on their babies' bodies, who were often struggling physically before receiving donor milk, but transformed within a few days of consuming it. Shirley had low milk supply with her first child, Benjamin, and experienced difficulties again with her second child, Vivian. A few days after Vivian's birth, Shirley could tell she was not doing well. She explained, "Her jaundice was not going away. She had a bunch of extra jaundice and her poor face was purple from birth. She was starting to get lethargic and she hadn't had any poop." Shirley called her midwife, Rose, who worked at Holistic Health and gave her Sara's phone number to call for milk. It was Mother's Day when Shirley called Sara to explain her circumstances and ask her for milk. Shirley explained that during the conversation, "I completely fell apart with a stranger on the phone. I'm like, 'It's Mother's Day and I can't feed my baby!'" Sara was also having a difficult Mother's Day, as she was in bed feeling sick from mastitis. The two had a great conversation, and Sara gave Shirley 150 ounces of milk later that day.

Shirley observed changes in Vivian after only a couple days of feeding her Sara's milk:

> 'So, my husband and I drove down right away and picked up the milk. We started supplementing and of course she rallied. The jaundice went away, and she was like a little wilted flower that perked back up. It was beautiful. It was just so good to see a healthy baby.'

Observed changes in the health status of recipient babies provides tangible evidence of the effectiveness of donated breastmilk (Falls 2017). These changes confirm the bio-intimate relationship between donor and recipient baby, demonstrating that the donor's bio-material transforms the baby's physical health and wellbeing. Expressions of gratitude based on the observed effects of donor milk on recipient babies were common, and donors felt pride and a sense of accomplishment when recipient caregivers shared photos of their thriving babies. Some recipients posted photos on social media sites, and others contacted donors directly to acknowledge them.

Grateful for the changes she saw in Vivian, Shirley sent Sara a text.

> 'I texted her and was like, "Thank you so much!" I was just gushing and so happy that my baby had rallied, and that really helps you to accept your breastfeeding situation when you see that your daughter is now pooping and smiling and hydrated and not jaundiced anymore. So, I thanked her, and she was like, "That is the nicest thing anybody has ever said to me." I was like, "Surely that's not the nicest thing, come on now." And she was like, "Actually, you're the only person who has thanked me." And I was like, "What? You're giving my daughter nourishment. *You* are responsible for my daughter thriving. What do you mean I'm the only person who's ever thanked you for that?" You know, because to me, there is no gift that you can give me that is as meaningful as breastmilk because I know the value of breastmilk. It is just this tremendous gift. I cannot imagine somebody not showing her gratitude, especially knowing what it takes to pump and to deal with all of that.'

Shirley recognized the connection between Vivian's health and Sara's milk as she watched Vivian's health transform. She acknowledged the bio-intimacy between the two, crediting Sara for Vivian's thriving health. Shirley continued:

> 'Of course, Sara won't take any credit for it, but I'm always like, "Look, you're growing this baby!" And the other day she kissed Vivian on the cheek, and she was like, "Oh, I'm sorry! I probably shouldn't just kiss your baby without permission." And I'm like, "Kiss her, she's half yours!" And I feel such gratitude towards her, so I'm glad that I get to have a friendship with my milk donor. It is still really hard for me to accept that I can't exclusively breastfeed Vivian myself, but again I'm super-grateful that I have this gorgeous, chubby, thriving baby. It's like, I'm so happy to have such a healthy baby that I'm okay with it. It just makes me feel so grateful. So sometimes I feel like I kind of try to generate a connection between Sara and Vivian. When we're together, I'm fine telling her, "She's half yours," you know what I mean? Just joking with her like that. And

> she of course will have nothing of that and is very humble about it. She was like, "I'm not up at the crack of dawn," you know, "I'm not up at four in the morning feeding her. So, don't say that. You're the mom." To her, it's just not a big deal. To me it's like, you've given my child health.'

From Shirley's perspective, the vitality that Sara provides for Vivian warranted a special social relationship between the two. Despite some level of connectedness, as evident in Sara's display of affection toward Vivian, Sara invoked broader cultural notions of family boundaries by minimizing her impact on Vivian's wellbeing and asserting that Shirley is Vivian's one and only mother. This negotiating of boundaries in the social relationships between donors and recipient children was common throughout our study, particularly in scenarios when donors and recipient caregivers established their own close relationships.

Later in the interview, Shirley drew a more distinct boundary between Sara as milk donor and herself as mother. For her, feeding Sara's milk to Vivian created a bio-intimate relationship between the two that warranted a special social connection, yet direct breastfeeding would have created a deeper level of intimacy that was beyond Shirley's comfort zone.

> 'I think wet nursing would be a lot harder for me. My milk donor, one time we talked about going to Disney together and she said something like, "Well, you wouldn't have to bring all that stuff, you have your milk donor right here." And she kind of offered, like she'd be open to cross-nursing. But I really don't think I would. No. And I'm so glad that we have pumps and whatnot because it would be extremely hard on me personally to see my daughter nursing from somebody else. I don't think I could handle it. There's such a connection between me and my daughter and even with all of the plastic that's involved, nursing is still really special. It's such a deep bond that I have with her that it would be really hard on me to let someone else nurse her. I mean, obviously if it were 200 years ago, and we didn't have a breast pump and whatever, I would rather have a living child. So, you know, it would have been a very different consideration. And then I would have been like, "Please, feed my baby." But now I wouldn't do that unless I was in some horrible circumstance. The emotional

> cost, I think, is huge because she's *my* baby to nurse. She's my baby to nurse.'

In this example, Shirley is comfortable recognizing Sara's contribution to Vivian's health and development, yet there are limits to the extent of physical and emotional connection she is willing to promote between the two. Asserting that Vivian is "my baby to nurse" reinforces the notion that breastfeeding is an intimate practice and draws on broader notions of neoliberal parenthood to construct the mother–child relationship as the ideal context for this level of intimacy. Shirley acknowledges that she would allow someone else to feed Vivian if it were necessary, but she is grateful for current technologies that facilitate donor breastmilk feeding without direct interembodied contact.

Sara did not mention her connection with Vivian during her interview but focused instead on the friendship she built with Shirley through sharing her milk. It is clear that she had a relationship with Vivian, evidenced by her kissing Vivian on the cheek, but this relationship was not a central component of milk sharing for Sara. Other donors felt a strong, parent-like sense of social connectedness to the children who consumed their breastmilk. Christine explained, "I feel like I have more of a connection with the baby. Not like when they're older I would say, 'Hey, I gave you breastmilk when you were a baby!' But almost like you feel like you have a part in the child's life, in the parenting, in the involvement and stuff."

Bio-connectedness

Although recipient caregivers do not establish bio-intimate relationships with donors since they do not consume the milk themselves, they are nevertheless connected through milk because of their interactions with it. Recipient caregivers make decisions about milk sharing, acquire milk from donors, transport, store and prepare it, and ultimately feed it to their children. They are integral to the practice of milk sharing, as they handle and manage the milk. Although they do not share bio-intimacy with donors, there is a bio-connectedness between the two, as the recipient caregiver moderates the transfer of biological material from the donor to the recipient child. Recipient caregivers handle and manage donors' biomaterial, make decisions about its use, and ascribe meaning to it. In so doing, they facilitate and moderate the bio-intimate relationships between donors and their children and create their own bio-connected relationships with donors.

For some donors and recipient caregivers, sharing milk was the basis of deep, personal friendships. Shirley and Sara developed a close, intimate friendship through their ongoing milk-sharing relationship. Shirley described her relationship with Benjamin's donor as more of a professional one, where they became Facebook friends, "but it's not like I was her BFF [best friend forever]". She was pleasantly surprised when she and Sara formed a friendship. She explained how their friendship developed after she sent Sara the text thanking her for her milk and describing how it had transformed Vivian:

> 'Then of course we started that conversation and we continued a friendship and we truly have continued to be friends. I'm happy to be her friend and it's really cool. I mean, you talked about screening the milk, and it's like, now we've been in each other's homes and we're close and we know each other's life story now and that sort of thing. It's really sweet and I'm glad that we have developed a friendship through all of that. I don't think a whole lot of people get to do that, and I'm so grateful for all of it. I am so glad that I have a local mom who was prescreened through my midwife that I was able to connect to and now I have a friendship with her.'

Sara also highlighted her friendship with Shirley during her interview:

> 'So, my exclusive, like my number one, she's pretty much my best friend. We met through Holistic Health, when she called me on Mother's Day hysterically crying, and she's my best friend now. We talk a lot. I don't think I've gone a day without talking to her since we've started. We just connected on a personal level. You know, she was a new mom, I was a new mom. I didn't really have a lot of friends locally and neither did she. We were both kind of newer to the area and so we just connected. The other moms I donate to, I have a few that I'm friends with on Facebook. There are others I've never met because I donated through Holistic Health, and I have a few that, especially when I first was donating, a few that would just text me when they needed milk.'

The kind of close personal friendship that developed between Sara and Shirley was not an automatic outcome of milk sharing, but it is not uncommon among people who share milk (Thorley 2012; Falls 2017; Gribble 2018; Wilson 2018). For those who developed close friendships and engaged in continuous, prolonged contact, there were opportunities for closer social relationships between the donor and recipient child. Within these relationships, the social meanings of the bio-intimate connections between donor and recipient child were negotiated.

Other participants also described establishing close kin-like relationships as a result of milk sharing. Jackie, a mother of four children who had always struggled to maintain a milk supply while working full time as a receptionist at a veterinarian clinic, was determined to breastfeed her youngest child, Addison. Natalie, a doctor at the vet clinic where Jackie worked, gave birth around the same time, and the two would pump milk together during breaks at work. After futile attempts to help Jackie express more milk through pumping, Natalie offered to provide breastmilk for Addison. Jackie explained:

> 'I have four daughters, my last one turned 11 months yesterday. I always struggled with breastfeeding and pumping and continuing to work and breastfeeding, so I made it my passion and that was my goal with this last baby that I was going to continue to breastfeed her. So, I went to work and luckily one of the doctors that I worked with was also pregnant, and she had a baby two weeks after me. She was also breastfeeding, pumping at work, so that support really helped. But I still didn't react well to a pump, so I was starting to struggle, and she could tell I was really frustrated. And so, one day she offered, she said she had an oversupply, and that she had milk she would offer. And because I knew her really well, I had worked with her for a while, I knew her history, I knew how healthy she was, and I trusted taking her milk.'

After some time, Natalie moved to another practice, but she continued giving breastmilk for Addison. Jackie would drive to Natalie's home, which was about an hour away, once a month to pick up milk. These pick-ups became social occasions, where the children and adults would spend time together. Jackie continued, "Since she started helping,

Figure 5.1: Connected by milk

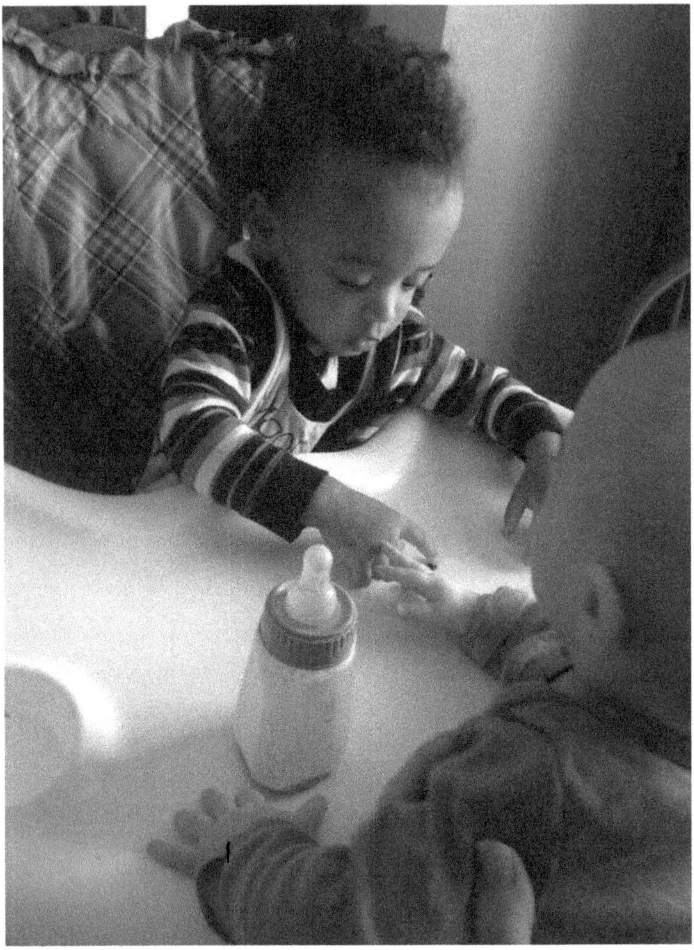

Source: Courtesy of Brittany Howell

there's just been a stronger bond between us and between our kids. We're like a family, it seems like" (Fig. 5.1).

Jackie described the human relationships that emerge through milk sharing as being "like a family", highlighting the feelings of connection and intimacy developed through the practice of sharing milk (Thorley 2012; Falls 2017; Gribble 2018; Wilson 2018). The social bonding is not just between Natalie and Addison, but includes Jackie and Natalie's children, who have all formed family-like relationships. She does not consider milk sharing actually making them family but uses the concept of family to emphasize the level of intimacy in their connection. Although milk sharing and some reproductive technologies have the capacity to transgress traditional definitions of family (Wilson 2018), as Kroløkke and Peterson (2017) point out, intimate social relationships are not automatically created by the transfer of biological material from one body to another, but instead are shaped by dominant social scripts that may be reproduced, challenged, or disrupted depending on the institutional and interpersonal context. To the predominantly white, cisgender, heterosexual milk-sharing participants we observed, the bio-intimate relationships created by milk sharing were special, and they created a sense of connection and intimacy, but they did not transgress family boundaries.

For others, milk sharing did not lead to close friendships, yet there was still a sense of connectedness. Nicole donated her milk to Laura, who had adopted a baby, Riley, and despite Laura's efforts, she was unable to induce lactation. Nicole described their relationship:

> 'I'm not close with Laura or anything, but I pumped for her for six months. She would bring Riley every time that we'd meet and so I'd get to see her grow and everything. She was so tiny at first, and Laura would send me pictures of her drinking my milk and it was so amazing to watch her grow. It was nice to get pictures of her. It just made me feel awesome. You can't explain that. I mean, to some other mom this is the best thing ever, to be able to feed her baby breastmilk. So, to me it was almost like a high to see a picture of a baby drinking your milk and you know that it made the mom's whole day, just to feed her that bottle.'

Although Nicole did not establish a close relationship with Laura or Riley, she appreciated seeing pictures of Riley drinking her milk and enjoyed watching her grow over the course of their milk-sharing relationship. Seeing the effects of her milk provided a strong sense of satisfaction, not only for the effects it had on Riley, but also because of the joy she knew it brought to Laura. This ability to use her biological material to help another mother nourish her baby, and to watch that baby grow, was "indescribable". Despite such strong positive feelings, bio-intimate relationships did not automatically generate close emotional relationships between the donor and recipient parent or child, as Nicole stated that she did not build close social relationships with her recipients. Nevertheless, she expressed a special sense of connectedness to Laura through their mutual contribution to Riley's healthy development and wellbeing.

In some instances, not feeling a connection to potential donors was a rationale for declining to receive milk. When Shirley received milk for her first child, Benjamin, she identified a potential donor, but when she arrived at the donor's home to pick up the milk, something didn't feel right. Shirley explained, "She seemed very different and very kind of off. It was awkward, and I don't know how to explain it." The donor had already packed up the milk in a cooler bag with dry ice, so Shirley felt obligated to take it. Once she arrived home, she defrosted one of the bags to inspect the milk, ultimately deciding not to feed it to Benjamin. She explained, "I think there was lipase[3] in the milk because it smelled a little funky and there was something about it. I don't know why I just didn't feel right. And I didn't have that connection with her." After consulting her midwife, Shirley decided not to feed the milk to Benjamin, but she found another milk recipient who felt comfortable with the milk, despite Shirley's full disclosure, so she passed it on. While Shirley rejected the milk due to her concerns about its safety, her lack of connection with the donor initiated her suspicion towards the milk. Thus, in some instances, a sense of interpersonal connection between the donor and recipient caregiver is important for trusting the quality of the milk. A recipient caregiver who does not trust a donor will likely refuse to facilitate a bio-intimate relationship between that donor and their child. In this way, trust is a central aspect of milk sharing (Cassidy 2012a, 2012b; Gribble 2014a, 2014c, 2018; Palmquist 2015; Falls 2017; Shaw and Morgan 2017; Carter et al 2018; Reyes-Foster and Carter 2018a, 2018b).

In other instances, donors may refuse to give milk to potential recipients based on lack of connections with them, or questions about their motives (Gribble 2014b; Reyes-Foster and Carter 2018a, 2018b). Cassie refused to give her milk to a potential recipient because she thought the recipient was hiding milk sharing from her husband. Cassie was one of only two donors we interviewed who donated and sold milk. Cassie used various websites to identify recipients and buyers, was a member of several private Facebook groups for women who breastfeed and donate milk, and served as moderator of a well-known national breastfeeding group for a few years. She explained that because she found many of her recipients through the internet, many of whom were not local to Florida, she screened them to protect herself from "scams", which could be someone trying to obtain milk to resell it, or a man using human milk to aid in body building.[4] Because she viewed her milk as precious, she wanted to make sure it would be used to nourish a baby, even when she sold it. Cassie explained:

> 'There was a woman a few months ago who had contacted me and something all along had felt funny about her. Towards the end we had agreed to how much milk she wanted and she informed me that she wanted me to ship it to a different address than her PayPal address because she didn't want her husband to know. I told her that I wasn't comfortable with that because she was hiding it from him. The fact was that she was hiding it because he was uncomfortable about the idea about milk sharing and she was trying not to let him know that she was receiving this milk from someone. So, I just had to tell her that I appreciated her desire to feed her child in that way, but I wasn't comfortable. So, it was just something that to me wasn't in my comfort zone. I had to tell her no just because of that.'

Cassie's refusal to sell her breastmilk to a mother hiding the practice from her husband reflects the interplay between the intimacy of milk sharing and issues of consent. Informed consent is an important component of the use of human milk in hospital settings, which is obtained through a formal process of explaining the risks and benefits to parents, often repositioning milk from human bodily fluid to a healing substance akin to medicine (Carroll 2014). Because peer milk sharing takes place without any formal, institutional oversight, there are no specific protocols that must be followed regarding informed consent. Instead, consent is negotiated by individuals in context. Consent can often be assumed by a potential recipient requesting milk or accepting it, which, in many cases, is enacted by a recipient child's mother. Fathers, spouses and other parenting partners typically provided informal consent by supporting the mothers' decisions to engage in milk sharing, and some picked up milk from donors' homes and fed the milk to their children, even when they were initially "grossed out" by the idea of using someone else's milk. Other researchers have documented some instances where breastmilk has been fed to babies without any parental consent, sometimes resulting in public controversy (Giles 2003; Shaw 2004a, 2007). Without a protocol to follow, Cassie drew on hegemonic definitions of family to inform her decision to refuse providing milk without the full consent of the recipient's spouse. She rejected forming bio-intimate and bio-connected relationships with this family in the absence of informed consent.

This chapter has explored the interconnectedness of milk-sharing bio-communities of practice. By describing the foundational context from which milk sharing emerges and the ways in which milk-sharing participants connect with each other through discourse, practice and milk, we demonstrate how bio-communities of practice are operationalized. We also illuminate how individuals are connected through biological materials. Whereas bio-communities are connected through practice, individuals who are connected through milk experience bio-intimacy and bio-connectedness. In Chapter 2, we described how milk is a living, agentive material full of emotive value, and in Chapter 4 we demonstrated how the labour involved in its production plays a key role in its value. In this chapter, we have illustrated how global and local forces come together to create the context and connections necessary for milk sharing to not only exist but thrive.

6

Conclusion

As we approached the final chapter of this book, two news headlines were circulating within the milk-sharing communities we studied. The first, an article in *The Washington Post* titled "Why These Bikers Crisscross New York Delivering Donated Breast Milk" (Free 2019), tells the heartwarming story of a motorcycle club that has partnered with an HMBANA milk bank in New York to deliver pasteurized breastmilk to homes and hospitals for babies who need it. The article emphasizes the altruism in both breastmilk donation and delivery by the motorcyclists, showing how two unlikely worlds – motorcycling and breastmilk feeding – come together for a greater purpose. The milk is referred to as 'precious cargo', and its health benefits to the receiving babies are presented as scientifically indisputable. The article emphasizes the social relationships that emerge from the partnership, where the motorcyclists connect with the founder of the milk bank as well as the parents and babies to whom they bring milk. These community connections, along with the greater purpose of delivering human milk to needy babies, is described as 'wonderful', 'rewarding' and 'inspired by kindness'.

The second headline derives from a news article from *Physician's Weekly* titled "AAP: Most Moms Unconcerned with Informal Milk Sharing" (HealthDay News 2019). The article reports a new study presented at the American Academy of Pediatrics annual meeting that used survey data to assess concerns related to breastmilk obtained through 'informal milk sharing' rather than through milk banks. The article reports that a high percentage of participants who used peer-shared milk were not concerned about the quality of the milk, and most did not screen donors because they trusted them. These findings are presented as problematic, and cause for serious concern. The article characterizes peer milk in terms of risk, stating that peer milk sharing is 'discouraged by the pediatric medical community'. It concludes with a quote from one of the researchers, stating that it is 'crucial that physicians become aware of this practice and the associated risks so that they can educate patients and address this growing concern'.

These articles reflect an ongoing cultural narrative that presents the use of banked breastmilk as safe, medically supported, and contributing to a greater moral good, and the use of peer breastmilk as risky, medically discouraged, and an emergent social problem. Peer milk recipients are consistently portrayed as naïve for failing to engage in diligent screening procedures (Carter et al 2015). When the second article was shared on Facebook by Madeline, a midwife who facilitates peer milk sharing through the Holistic Health Birth Center, the responses corroborated our research findings. Madeline wrote at the top of her post, 'Thoughts? If you don't know a donor do you request labs?' Some participants responded that they would never accept milk from someone they didn't know personally, as such sharing would be 'very, very risky in my opinion'. Some responded by citing the importance of donor screening, and shared information about how they implemented it in their own milk-sharing practices. Others who were donors described the medical screenings they had prior to donating, and the care they took in producing, handling and labelling their milk. One donor concluded, 'I took it seriously. I would never give someone else's baby something I wouldn't give my own.'

Stories like these and the conversations that ensue around them on social media are part of the foundational context from which milk sharing emerges. In our prior work (Carter et al 2015; Carter and Reyes-Foster 2016), we have identified ways that milk banking and milk sharing are differentially portrayed in public discourse, and we have also analyzed how women who engage in milk sharing consume and interpret these messages (Reyes-Foster and Carter 2018c). It came as no surprise to us that a paediatric researcher would find that women who engage in 'informal' milk sharing would be unconcerned with its safety: cumulative social science knowledge of peer milk sharing shows that on-the-ground practices do not align with how milk sharing is understood by some biomedical researchers and professional organizations and government entities such as the AAP and the USFDA (Gribble 2013, 2014a; Palmquist and Doehler 2014, 2016; Stuebe et al 2014; Reyes-Foster et al 2015; Falls 2017; Carter et al 2018; Reyes-Foster and Carter 2018c; Wilson 2018; Palmquist et al 2019). Thus, when milk-sharing participants consume discourses about peer milk sharing in public media, they are more likely to be skeptical of alarmist reports that cast milk sharing as unsafe. In this book, we have sought to make a timely intervention into this topic as a way of bridging the gap of understanding between members of the medical community and the popular press, which continues to propagate a misinformed understanding of peer milk sharing.

Summary of the book

Throughout this book, we have provided a detailed analysis of how peer milk sharing takes place on the ground, illuminating the reasons parents and other caregivers engage in the practice, the meanings they attribute to it, and the relationships they develop in the process. We focused our research on a single locale over a several year period to facilitate a holistic understanding of the multiple forms milk sharing takes, enabling us to illustrate patterns that develop in both online and offline environments. In so doing, we demonstrate how the broader natural and mainstream childbirth and parenting discourses, along with the social networks, healthcare providers, and consumer products they correspond with, provide the foundational context from which peer milk sharing emerges. The most significant element of this foundational context is breastfeeding promotion, where expectant parents learn about the nutritional and immunological benefits of breastmilk and are convinced that they should make breastfeeding a priority (Wall 2001; Kukla 2006; Wolf 2007, 2010; Crossley 2009; Jansson 2009; Knaak 2010; Waggoner 2011). Although most US mothers initiate breastfeeding, many experience physical and social obstacles that prevent them from meeting their breastfeeding goals, and for those who become parents through adoption, surrogacy, or other means, breastfeeding is most often not a viable option (Kelleher 2006; Lee 2007, 2008; Marshall et al 2007; Zizzo 2011; Cross-Barnet et al 2012; Stearns 2013; Wilson 2018). The existence and growing popularity of human milk banks – as well as bioventure capitalist efforts to commodify human milk through technological processing – provide a form of medically sanctioned human milk sharing that formally designates human milk from an unrelated individual as a superior alternative to infant formula (Bar-Yam 2010; Hassan 2010). Within this cultural milieu, peer milk-sharing organizations and informal networks also exist, comprising maternity and infant healthcare providers who support milk sharing, donors and recipients who engage in it, and leaders of organizations that facilitate milk sharing such as Get Pumped and Human Milk 4 Human Babies (Cassidy 2012a, 2012b; Gribble 2013; Perrin et al 2014, 2018; Palmquist 2015; Falls 2017; Shaw and Morgan 2017; Palmquist et al 2019). Collectively, these networks comprise global and local milk-sharing bio-communities of practice.

Within this broader cultural context, we have illustrated various paths through which individuals enter and become participants of milk-sharing bio-communities of practice. Many who become donors conform to the common media portrayal of breastfeeding mothers who have abundant milk, but others intended to give before they knew whether or not they would have any extra, and many became donors based on a personal request from a friend or someone in their broader online or offline social networks. Like donors in other studies (Falls 2017; Gribble 2018; Wilson 2018), some gave whatever excess milk they had only a few times, but others established elaborate pumping and feeding routines that enabled them to sustain long-term milk sharing relationships. Either way, donors engaged in significant body work and embodied labour to manage the quality and quantity of their milk, and physical labour to express, handle, store and transfer it. This extensive labour, along with donors' altruistic intentions and the vitality of human milk (Carroll 2014, 2015; Falls 2017; Shaw and Morgan 2017; Oreg 2019; Shaw 2019), contribute to the milk's emotive value. Peer-shared milk is valued for its health-giving properties, for the work that goes into its production, and for the desire to help that motivates its production. Human milk that is for sale is often viewed with suspicion, making peer milk a priceless gift but a worthless commodity (Hassan 2010; Gaard 2013; Shaw 2015, 2019; Falls 2017; Lee 2019). These common practices, and the values and norms that underlie them, are legitimized, sometimes contested, and reproduced in the physical and virtual spaces where milk sharing takes place.

Most who became peer milk recipients had either adopted or fostered babies or were mothers who were committed to breastfeeding but experienced difficulties producing enough to exclusively feed their own breastmilk, similar to recipients in other studies (Thorley 2012; Gribble 2013, 2014c; Palmquist and Doehler 2014, 2016; Palmquist 2015; Falls 2017; Wilson 2018). Some were transmasculine or gender non-binary who did not wish to breastfeed or had breastfeeding difficulties (MacDonald et al 2016; Giles 2017; Wilson 2018), and we encountered a few instances of maternal illness or death. Some recipients decided ahead of time that they would seek donor milk, but for others becoming a recipient was intertwined with an emotionally and physically challenging process of experiencing breastfeeding difficulties and ultimately recognizing that exclusive breastfeeding was not an option. Many participants learned about peer milk sharing during these difficult moments from the healthcare professionals, peers in breastfeeding support groups, and friends and family members who were supporting their breastfeeding efforts. On deciding to become a breastmilk recipient, they typically engaged in extensive, continual labour to identify and screen donors, procure their milk, store and handle it properly, feed it to their babies, and monitor their babies' responses to it. The positive effects recipient caregivers observed in their babies motivated them to continue seeking human milk (Falls 2017).

The sharing of human milk not only contributes to infant feeding, but also fosters interpersonal connectedness (Cassidy and El Tom 2010; Cassidy 2012a, 2012b; Shaw 2015, 2019; Falls 2017; Shaw and Morgan 2017; Gribble 2018; Lee 2018a). Individuals across the world who engage in peer milk sharing are connected by practice in global and local contexts (Cassidy and El Tom 2010; Cassidy 2012a, 2012b; Gribble 2014a, 2014b, 2018; Shaw and Morgan 2017; Shaw 2019). Local bio-communities of practice is where direct milk sharing most often takes place, as individuals connect with others through their local online and offline social networks to learn and share information about milk sharing, identify potential donors or recipients, and ultimately, share milk. These local communities converge on a global level as individuals engage in similar practices that are motivated by their commitment to breastmilk feeding and a collective orientation toward it. They share representations of milk sharing on social media, educating others about it, and reinforcing the values and ideals that support it. Whereas all who participate in peer milk sharing are connected through practice, donor–recipient pairs who share milk directly are connected through milk. Donors and the children who consume their milk share bio-intimacy, as the donor's biological material enters and transforms the recipient child's body (Falls 2017; Shaw and Morgan 2017; Shaw 2019). Donors and recipient caregivers share bio-connectedness, as recipient caregivers moderate the transfer of biological material from donor to recipient child, and they handle and manage the milk. To some, bio-intimacy and bio-connectedness are a foundation for deep, kin-like relationships. To others, milk sharing is part of a more personal journey to feed their own babies breastmilk or to give milk to others.

Informing policy and practice

Scientific debates regarding the safety of peer milk sharing have been contentious and no consensus has been reached. A research team led by Sarah Keim (Keim et al 2013, 2015) tested and found unsafe levels of bacteria and traces of cow's milk in breastmilk purchased online and shipped through the mail. This study has implications for the use of breastmilk acquired through these means, but as this book has demonstrated and consistent with other studies of how peer milk sharing takes place (Gribble 2013, 2014a, 2018; Palmquist and Doehler 2014, 2016; Falls 2017; Wilson 2018), the practices used by Keim and colleagues to collect breastmilk are not reflective of how parents and other caregivers acquire human milk to feed their babies. Their samples were collected from strangers through the milk-selling website Only the Breast, without any further interaction or screening beyond the original request to purchase the milk and directions on where to ship it. Our research and that of others has shown that most recipients engage in some form of donor screening (Gribble 2014a; Palmquist and Doehler 2016; Falls 2017; Reyes-Foster et al 2017), and that strangers are often screened more rigorously than friends, family members, or those identified through healthcare providers or other close social networks. Participants meet in person to transfer the milk, which is also part of the screening process. Taboos against the sale of breastmilk reveal that many milk-sharing participants are as skeptical of commodified human milk as Keim's research team and the public health officials who warn against buying milk over the internet (Cassidy 2012a; Gribble 2013, 2014a, 2014b, 2014c, 2018; Palmquist and Doehler 2014, 2016; Falls 2017; Shaw and Morgan 2017; Wilson 2018; Shaw 2019). Keim's research is therefore unable to speak to the healthiness and safety of the human milk shared in the ways we and other social scientists have documented (Perrin et al 2018; Palmquist et al 2019).

More recently, ethnographically informed biomedical research that takes known practices of peer milk sharing into account in study design has been published in one study to date (Perrin et al 2018). In their research, Maryanne T. Perrin and colleagues found no significant differences in the nutritional composition and bacterial content between mothers' own, banked, peer-shared, and professionally screened breastmilk. Moreover, contrary to findings in research on purchased human milk, the researchers found no evidence of adulteration or water dilution. Perrin and colleagues conclude, 'These findings are contrary to findings of risks in paid models of human milk exchange and fill an important gap in the scientific literature for health care providers and families seeking evidence regarding risks and benefits of peer-to-peer milk sharing' (2018: 9). More studies like that of Perrin and colleagues, alongside social scientific research, are needed for public health and biomedical organizations to make evidence-based recommendations regarding the use of peer-shared milk. It could be the case that all of the forms of milk sharing we have described here result in infant-feeding methods that are more or less safe and healthy when compared with infant formula feeding, or perhaps there are some milk-sharing practices that are superior and others that are inferior. More research testing the safety and healthiness of milk shared in various forms that reflect actual practices is needed to answer these questions.

After years of calling for more biomedical research into the safety of peer milk sharing, Perrin and colleagues' (2018) study, which has groundbreaking methods, findings and implications, received little attention from the media. Where Keim's study that found bacteria in milk bought online was featured in many news stories, even appearing on the cover of the Sunday *New York Times* in 2013, Perrin and colleagues' research received little coverage from news media. In contrast, media coverage of preliminary findings of a newer study that again casts peer milk sharing in a negative light and were only reported in an oral presentation at a medical conference was widespread, with the story appearing on myriad highly trafficked online sources such as the pregnancy website The Bump, Technology Networks, the AAP website and Science Friday. It is unfortunate that alarmist research findings continue to hold greater sway and staying power than sound scientific research. In this book, we aim to present a nuanced understanding of peer milk sharing, and although we recognize our collective work in capturing the attention of biomedical researchers and policymakers is far from done, we shall continue to collaborate with our colleagues working in this area towards a goal of better informed public discourses of peer milk sharing.

Evidence-based public discourses of peer milk sharing are important because, as we demonstrate in this book, those who participate in breastmilk sharing engage with dominant biomedical messaging regarding infant feeding, taking away the message that 'breast is best, donor next'. This interpretation emerges from a foundational context that contains contradictory messages, where parents are educated on the benefits of breastmilk and the corresponding 'risks' associated with infant formula by healthcare providers, self-help maternity and childrearing literature, and dominant public health discourses (Wall 2001; Kukla 2006; Jansson 2009; Wolf 2010; Lee 2011; Waggoner 2011; Carter 2017). Through information shared by maternity care providers and peers over the internet, our participants interpret the WHO (2002) recommendations for infant feeding worldwide as recommending peer breastmilk over infant formula. While this interpretation is not entirely incongruent with the WHO statement, neither does it necessarily reflect the sentiment of the authors, whose recommendations were intended for global feeding strategies and may have been tailored differently for parents in post-industrial societies. Certainly, US-based public health and medical organizations such as the USFDA (2010) and AAP (2012, 2017), and their French and Canadian counterparts (Gribble and Hausman 2012), have taken a prohibitionist stance against peer milk sharing in their official statements. However, these statements are not widely publicized, and many of our participants were unfamiliar with them. Instead, our participants engaged in peer milk sharing as a form of community health promotion that they believed, in varying degrees, was consistent with dominant infant-feeding recommendations. They read alarmist media coverage of milk sharing as misguided, irrelevant to the kind of milk sharing they engaged in.

These findings suggest a need for more clarity and consistency in public health recommendations. If human breastmilk really is best for human babies, public health and community resources should be allocated to identify ways to increase the supply of safe and healthy human milk and distribute it to infants whose parents are otherwise unable to provide it. Peer milk sharing offers this potential to increase the supply of human milk (Akre et al 2011; Perrin et al 2018). By illustrating the multiple forms that peer milk sharing takes in Central Florida, our research provides potential models for sustainable, potentially safe, forms of breastmilk sharing. Alternatively, if the benefits of breastmilk have been overstated, as Wolf (2010) argues, and biomedical research is able to show that infant formula feeding is actually safer and healthier than human milk shared in each of the forms identified through empirical research, this message needs to be conveyed and publicized in ways that are clear, consistent and evidence-based.

In conjunction with clearer public health messaging, new technological developments could provide possibilities for ensuring the safety of peer-shared milk. The development of home test strips that allow caregivers to test thawed milk for bacteria or other pathogens could alleviate many concerns held by public health officials about peer milk sharing. Such test strips would be useful not only for testing milk that is shared among peers, but also for ensuring that milk expressed for one's own infant has not been contaminated by improper or imperfect sterilization and milk-handling techniques. As 65% of mothers with young children work in the paid US labour force (United States Department of Labor 2018), many of those who breastfeed beyond the first few weeks of life rely on their own expressed milk as a central component of breastfeeding (Avishai 2004; Stearns 2010; Johnson and Salpini 2017; Johnson 2019). Many peer milk donors in our study had initially expressed the milk they donated for their own babies, only later identifying that they had more than they needed, which they gave to a peer recipient. The logic we heard from many donors and recipients alike is that if a bottle of milk is healthy for a mother's own baby, why wouldn't that same bottle of milk be healthy for someone else's baby? These concerns over contamination could be mitigated with the development of affordable home test strips, ensuring that all expressed human milk fed to infants is safe.

The potential of human milk sharing

The potential of milk sharing lies in the underlying desire to build a world where all babies have access to human milk, which motivates donors and recipients to spend considerable effort in giving and seeking milk. And while these bio-communities of practice are homogenous in many respects, milk-sharing communities transcend other differences. In the communities we observed in Central Florida and those studied by others (for example, Falls 2017; Wilson 2018), milk sharing attracts people on opposite sides of political and religious spectrums. It brings together and sometimes facilitates long-lasting relationships between people who might otherwise never encounter each other and who might vehemently disagree on major questions of society and morality. As others who have studied the practice have noted (Falls 2017; Shaw and Morgan 2017; Lee 2018a; Wilson 2018; Shaw 2019), milk sharing reflects an alternative mode of being to the construct of the self-serving, bounded, highly individuated, neoliberal subject. It forces a recognition that even in contemporary societies in the Global North, human beings remain interconnected and interdependent. Milk sharing is driven by the shared belief that all babies deserve human milk and that human milk will directly benefit the babies who consume it. These babies will grow up and reap the social and physical benefits of the milk they were given as infants, affording them the potential to make the world a better place. Milk sharing is as much about the future as it is about the present.

Notes

Chapter 1

1 There are many pathways to becoming a breastfeeding educator or counsellor, requiring varied levels of training and education, which may result in titles such as Certified Lactation Counsellor, Certified Lactation Educator, Certified Lactation Specialist, Breastfeeding Counsellor and so on. In 1985, breastfeeding experts joined together from around the world to create a consistent set of qualifications for lactation specialists. The group created the International Board of Lactation Consultant Examiners to oversee and establish professional licensure for the new profession, known as International Board Certified Lactation Consultant (IBCLC). IBCLC certification requires 14 college-level courses in health sciences or related areas, 90 hours of lactation-specific coursework, 300–1,000 hours of clinical supervision, and passing a certification exam (Walker and Aldridge 2017).

2 For more on Get Pumped, visit http://getpumpedonline.org.

3 Here, we define a market as a space where the forces of supply and demand operate and buyers and sellers interact to trade goods, services, or instruments for money or barter.

4 We allowed individuals who had donated to a milk bank to complete the survey because many in the communities we studied considered Get Pumped to be a milk bank. Only five survey participants only ever donated to an HMBANA-affiliated milk bank. These participants were omitted from our analysis because they did not participate in peer breastmilk sharing.

5 This research was approved by the University of Central Florida office for the protection of human subjects (IRB Protocols SBE-14-10207 and SBE-15-11300).

6 For more information about the demographic characteristics of our sample and descriptive analyses of their milk-sharing and milk-handling practices, please see Reyes-Foster et al 2015 and 2017.

Chapter 2

1 This appears to be a common strategy, also described by Kristin Wilson (2018) and Susan Falls (2017).

2 Our survey research on human milk handling (Reyes-Foster, et al 2017) and our interviews suggests this is an unusual stance. In our survey data, respondents reported engaging in mostly safe milk-handling practices. Most of our interview participants described – and demonstrated, when we interviewed them at

home – elaborate food-handling practices and routines to reduce risk of bacterial contamination.

3 See Carter et al (2018) for more on this.

4 This perspective has, however, been critiqued (Brekke and Sirnes 2011).

5 We should note, however, that Plummer's work is tangential to Wilson's argument, which is primarily grounded in the New Materialisms and reproductive justice.

6 In the 1960s, when the legal status of banked blood was being defined, opponents of for-profit blood banking argued that treating blood as a commodity, thereby giving ownership rights to the people it came from, would produce waste. For instance, in the 1984 case Moore v. Regents of the University of California, John Moore, the plaintiff, argued that because he owned the spleen from which his physician had later created a lucrative immortal cell line he was entitled to part of the profits. In ruling for the defence, the court reasoned that 'without gifts of money and tissues from the public to researchers … the public would cease to receive improved medical products and therapies' (101). Thus, the reason blood and tissues were explicitly defined as gifts was not due to a bioethical prerogative, but rather to the legal disempowerment of the people from whom these substances were taken. While universities and corporations were able to patent stem lines created from tissues and profit from them, the people from whom these tissues were taken could not claim ownership over them in a court of law. In the Moore decision, the court suggested that tissue samples had to operate according to both the regime of the gift (in the free flow of information between scientists and institutions) and commodity (in the creation of products derived from the tissue that could be sold for profit).

7 Initially, one might think that human milk, because it 'is imbued with labor and love' (Wilson 2018: 4), is perhaps even more active and lively. However, a materialist approach will retort that 'labour' and 'love' are symbolic, rather than material, ways of understanding milk.

Chapter 3

1 A galactagogue is a substance that is understood to help increase breastmilk production. The most commonly used galactagogues are non-pharmaceutical, including foods and herbs. Although there are few scientific studies that adequately measure their effectiveness for increasing milk supply (Budzynska et al 2012), qualitative interview research with mothers who use them identifies themes of self-empowerment and confidence in relation to their ability to exclusively breastfeed (Sim et al 2015). Domperidone is a pharmaceutical medication that is a dopamine D_2 receptor antagonist, which is not USFDA-approved, but is approved in most other countries for treatment of nausea, vomiting and gastroparesis, a condition characterized by inability for the stomach to empty itself normally. Although it was not developed to aid lactation, Domperidone contributes to increased prolactin, which stimulates milk production. In clinical trials, Domperidone is found to significantly increase milk production in about two thirds of lactating mothers experiencing insufficient milk supply (Wan et al 2008). Domperidone was easily purchased from overseas among our study participants.

2 Necrotizing enterocolitis (NEC) is an extremely serious disease that affects mostly premature infants. Human milk has been demonstrated to reduce the risk of NEC (Hermann and Carroll 2014; Patel and Kim 2018).

3 A supplemental nursing system (SNS) is the Medela brand version of a supplemental feeding tube device (SFTD) in which supplemental milk (expressed breastmilk or formula) from a small container that hangs around the caregiver's neck is slowly released through a tube connected to the caregiver's nipple. SFTDs are used to stimulate milk production by the caregiver and promote skin-to-skin contact while keeping the nursling satisfied by receiving milk. SFTDs can be used temporarily to aid in establishing or re-establishing a caregiver's milk supply, or it can be used longer term in cases of adoptive nursing, breast reduction surgery, or insufficient milk supply (Borucki 2005).

4 Tongue-tie, the common term for ankyloglossia, is characterized by a short lingual frenulum, which can restrict movement of the tongue, causing poor latch and other breastfeeding problems. It can be corrected with frenotomy, which is a tongue-tie division procedure (Brookes and Bowley 2014). Lip-tie is characterized by attachment of the upper lip to the gingival tissue, which can restrict mobility and prevent the upper lip from properly flanging to create a good seal on the breast. Lip-tie can also be surgically released (Kotlow 2013).

Chapter 5

1 Midwives who work in out-of-hospital settings can only provide care to pregnant women who have low-risk pregnancies and do not experience certain complications during pregnancy or labour. Therefore, not everyone who seeks an out-of-hospital birth will have one, but finances are less commonly the primary barrier. In addition, not all midwifery practices are considered to be 'in-network' providers, so those with private insurance may encounter other costs, although the cost of a birth centre or home birth is significantly less than the cost of a hospital birth.

2 Insufficient glandular tissue (IGT), also referred to as mammary hypoplasia, is an uncommon condition in which women lack sufficient glandular tissue to produce sufficient milk, despite having normal hormone levels (Arbour and Kessler 2013).

3 Bile salt stimulated lipase (commonly referred to as 'lipase') is a bioactive protein in human breastmilk. Typically, it comprises 1–2% of the total milk proteins, and its function is to aid in the digestion of milk fat in the gut (Lönnerdal 2013). Refrigeration does not affect lipase activity, although it can be affected by freezing. For some mothers, typically those producing milk for older infants or toddlers, freezing milk may result in high lipase activity, which does not appear to have negative health consequences for infants consuming the milk, but can produce a 'soapy' or rancid odour and taste, causing some infants to refuse to drink it (Kim and Froh 2012).

4 There is a growing trend for men to use breastmilk to aid body building. Breastmilk donors tend to be opposed to this practice, often wanting to see evidence of a baby who will be consuming their milk before donating it. However, men who want it seem to be able to purchase milk via websites such as Only the Breast (Eidelman 2015; Lieber 2014). One participant in our study, Lisa, who donated milk through Only the Breast to a mother in Tennessee, charging only for the costs of shipping and dry ice, was contacted by a few men seeking to purchase her milk, requests that she declined.

Appendix A: Survey Participant Demographics

Table A.1 displays the demographic characteristics of survey participants. Participants consisted of 392 individuals who reported engaging in peer milk sharing. Demographic data show that nearly 90% of respondents were white. Most participants were college-educated, with 64.6% reporting a bachelor's degree or higher. The sample was also socioeconomically privileged: nearly half of participants reported household incomes above US$70,001 a year and nearly 25% reported incomes above US$100,000 per year. The most common employment status was 'not employed', indicating that respondents were likely raising small children at home with the financial support of a spouse, followed by 'employed full-time'. More than 70% of participants reported having only one or two children (see Table A.2). The majority identified as cisgender (99.7%) and heterosexual (95.3%). All but five of our respondents (99% of the sample) reported participating in peer breastmilk sharing since 2010, the year that Eats on Feets and Human Milk 4 Human Babies first appeared.

Table A.1: Survey participant demographics by type of milk sharing

	Donor only (N=240)	**Recipient only (N=83)**	**Donor and recipient (N=69)**
Race/ethnicity			
White	4.9%	7.8%	6.5%
Hispanic/Latino	89.3%	87.5%	88.7%
Black/African American	2.9%	0.0%	0.0%
Other	3.0%	4.7%	4.8%
Income level			
<$25,001	7.5%	7.8%	14.8%
$25,001–$55,000	29.7%	32.8%	23.0%
$55,001–$85,000	28.2%	26.5%	24.6%
$85,001–$100,000	11.0%	7.8%	11.5%
>$100,000	23.6%	25.0%	26.2%
Education level			
High school diploma or less	3.4%	9.2%	1.6%
Some college education or associate's degree	33.0%	30.8%	27.9%
Bachelor's degree	34.0%	29.2%	36.1%
Master's degree, doctorate degree or professional degree (MD or JD)	29.6%	30.8%	34.4%
Number of children			
1	43.7%	36.9%	25.8%
2	37.4%	47.7%	41.9%
3	14.6%	9.2%	19.4%
4 or more	4.4%	6.1%	13.0%
Employment status			
Full-time	40.8%	32.3%	35.5%
Part-time	14.1%	24.6%	21.0%
Not employed	45.1%	43.1%	43.5%
Sexual orientation			
Straight	96.4%	88.1%	96.9%
Gay/lesbian	0.5%	1.49%	0.0%
Bi-/multisexual	3.1%	10.5%	3.1%

Source: Reyes-Foster et al 2015

Appendix B: Interview Participant Demographics

Table A.2 displays the demographic characteristics of interview participants. Participants consisted of 30 individuals who resided in Central Florida and took part in peer milk sharing at the time of the interview. All identified as cisgender, heterosexual women. They were predominantly white, with two of the 30 identifying as white-Hispanic. They ranged in age from 20–45, with a median age of 30. With regard to marital status, 22 were married at the time of the interview, five were cohabiting with two of these five engaged to marry, two were single and one was divorced. Most participants had some college education, with six holding a master's degree or higher, six holding a bachelor's degree, 15 reporting some college education, an associate's degree, or current college enrolment at the time of interview, and two participants had a high school diploma or equivalent. Regarding income, 13 participants reported annual incomes lower than US$48,900, the median household income in Florida in 2015 (US Department of Labor 2018), with two reporting below the poverty threshold US Department of Labor 2018), whereas 17 participants reported annual incomes higher than the median, with four reporting incomes higher than $100,000. In terms of religious affiliation, 19 participants identified as Christian or as a particular Protestant sect such as Methodist, three identified as Catholic, one identified as Jewish, six reported no religious affiliation, and one reported being agnostic.

Table A.2: Interview participant demographics

Name	Age	Race/ Ethnicity	Education	Marital status	Religious affiliation	Household income*	Donor/ recipient
Alexa	36	White	Master's	Married	Methodist	$75,000	Donor
Allison	24	White	Associate's	Married	Christian	$60,000	Donor
Anna	21	White	Some college	Cohabiting/ engaged	Christian	$45,000	Recipient
Ashley	34	White	Some college	Married	Christian	$75,000	Donor
Cassie	29	White	Bachelor's	Married	Christian	$70,000	Donor
Christine	25	White	High school	Married	Christian	$30,000	Both
Crystal	36	White	Master's	Married	Christian	$37,500	Both
Elaine	42	White	Bachelor's	Married	None	$67,000	Donor
Emily	30	White	Some college	Cohabiting	Christian	$35,000	Donor
Georgianna	26	White	Bachelor's	Married	Christian	$34,000	Donor
Hope	21	White	Some college	Engaged	Catholic	$76,075	Donor
Ingrid	21	White	High School Equivalent	Married	Christian	$18,000	Donor
Isabella	33	White	Master's	Married	Christian	$110,000	Donor
Jackie	30	White	Some college	Married	None	$36,000	Recipient

(continued)

Table A.2: Interview participant demographics (continued)

Jane	29	White	Some college	Married	Agnostic	$35,000	Donor
Janet	36	White-Hispanic	Master's	Married	Christian	$55,000	Donor
Kelly	26	White	In college	Cohabiting	None	$25,000	Donor
Lindsey	27	White	Associate's	Married	Methodist	$35,000	Donor
Lisa	30	White	Some college	Cohabiting	Catholic	$25,000	Donor
Louise	30	White	Some college	Married	None	$65,000	Donor
Mona Lisa	33	White/ Hispanic	Master's	Single	Christian	$50,000	Recipient
Nicole	20	White	Associate's	Divorced	Christian	$20,000	Donor
Olivia	45	White	Master's	Single	None	$40,000	Recipient
Raven	29	White	Trade school	Married	None	$50,000	Donor
Rhonda	40	White	Bachelor's	Married	Catholic	$80,000	Recipient
Sara	28	White	Bachelor's	Married	Jewish	$100,000	Donor
Samantha	32	White	Bachelor's	Married	Anglican	$125,000	Both
Shirley	32	White	Bachelor's	Married	Christian	$60,000	Recipient
Thelma	29	White	Some college	Married	Christian	$125,000	Recipient
Trisha	30	White	Associate's	Married	Christian	$56,000	Donor

* Participants provided an estimate of household income. For those who provided a range, we report the median.

References

AAN (American Academy of Nursing). (2016). "Position Statement Regarding Use of Informally Shared Human Milk." *Nursing Outlook* 64(1):98–102.

AAP (American Academy of Pediatrics). (2012). "Breastfeeding and the Use of Human Milk." *Pediatrics* 129(3):e827-e41.

AAP. (2017). "Donor Human Milk for the High-Risk Infant: Preparation, Safety, and Usage Options in the United States. Policy Statement." *Pediatrics* 139(1):e20163440.

ABM (Academy of Breastfeeding Medicine). (2010). "ABM Clinical Protocol #8: Human Milk Storage Information for Home Use for Full-Term Infants." *Breastfeeding Medicine* 5(3):127–30.

Afflerback, Sara, Amanda Koontz Anthony, Shannon K. Carter and Liz Grauerholz. (2014)."Consumption Rituals in the Transition to Motherhood." *Gender Issues* 31(1):1–20.

Afflerback, Sara, Shannon K. Carter, Amanda Koontz Anthony and Liz Grauerholz. (2013). "Infant-Feeding Consumerism in the Age of Intensive Mothering and Risk Society." *Journal of Consumer Culture* 13(3):387–405.

Akre, James E., Karleen D. Gribble and Maureen Minchin. (2011). "Milk Sharing: From Private Practice to Public Pursuit." *International Breastfeeding Journal* 6:8.

Al-Shehri, Saad S. et al. (2015). "Breastmilk-Saliva Interactions Boost Innate Immunity by Regulating the Oral Microbiome in Early Infancy." PloS ONE 10(9):e0135047.

Altorki, Soraya. (1980). "Milk-Kinship in Arab Society: An Unexplored Problem in the Ethnography of Marriage." *Ethnology* 19(2):233–44.

A Negro Nurse. (2001). "More Slavery at the South." *The Independent* 72:196–200.

Andrews, Therese and Stephanie Knaak. (2013). "Medicalized Mothering: Experiences with Breastfeeding in Canada and Norway." *The Sociological Review* 61(1):88–110.

Appadurai, Arjun. (1986). *The Social Life of Things: Commodities in Cultural Perspective*. Cambridge: Cambridge University Press.

Arbour, Megan W. and Julia Lange Kessler. (2013). "Mammary Hypoplasia: Not Every Breast Can Produce Sufficient Milk." *Journal of Midwifery & Women's Health* 58(4):457–61.

Arnold, Lois D.W. and Laraine Lockhart Borman. (1996). "What Are the Characteristics of the Ideal Human Milk Donor?" *Journal of Human Lactation* 12(2):143–45.

Asiodu, Ifeyinwa V., Catherine M. Waters, Dawn E. Dailey, Kathryn A. Lee and Audrey Lyndon. (2015). "Breastfeeding and Use of Social Media among First-Time African American Mothers." *Journal of Obstetric, Gynecologic & Neonatal Nursing* 44(2):268–78.

Avishai, Orit. (2004). "At the Pump." *Journal of the Motherhood Initiative for Research and Community Involvement* 6(2):139–49.

Avishai, Orit. (2007). "Managing the Lactating Body: The Breast-Feeding Project and Privileged Motherhood." *Qualitative Sociology* 30(2):135–52.

Avishai, Orit (ed). (2011). *Managing the Lactating Body: The Breastfeeding Project in the Age of Anxiety*. New York, NY: Springer.

Azema, Emilie and Stacey Callahan. (2003). "Breast Milk Donors in France: A Portrait of the Typical Donor and the Utility of Milk Banking in the French Breastfeeding Context." *Journal of Human Lactation* 19(2):199–202.

Ballard, Olivia and Ardythe L. Morrow. (2013). "Human Milk Composition: Nutrients and Bioactive Factors." *Pediatric Clinics of North America* 60(1):49–74.

Bartlett, Alison. (2002). "Breastfeeding as Headwork: Corporeal Feminism and Meanings for Breastfeeding." *Women's Studies International Forum* 25(3):373–82.

Bar-Yam, Naomi Bromberg. (2010). "The Story of the Mother's Milk Bank of New England." In Alison Bartlett and Rhonda Shaw (eds) *Giving Breastmilk: Body Ethics and Contemporary Breastfeeding Practices*. Bradford, Ontario: Demeter Press, pp. 98–109.

Bennett, Jane. (2010). *Vibrant Matter: A Political Ecology of Things*. Durham, NC: Duke University Press.

Berlant, Lauren. (2008). "Thinking about Feeling Historical." *Emotion, Space and Society* 1(1): 4–9.

Blum, Linda M. (1999). *At the Breast: Ideologies of Breastfeeding and Motherhood in the Contemporary United States*. Boston, MA: Beacon Press.

Blumer, Herbert. (1969). *Symbolic Interactionism: Perspective and Method*. Berkeley, CA: University of California Press.

Borucki, Lynne C. (2005). "Breastfeeding Mothers' Experiences Using a Supplemental Feeding Tube Device: Finding an Alternative." *Journal of Human Lactation* 21(4):429–38.

Boswell-Penc, Maia and Kate Boyer. (2007). "Expressing Anxiety? Breast Pump Usage in American Wage Workplaces." *Gender, Place and Culture* 14(5):551–67.

Bourdieu, Pierre. (1990). *The Logic of Practice*. Stanford, CA: Stanford University Press.

Bowman, Blythe. (2008). "Transnational Crimes Against Culture: Looting at Archaeological Sites and the 'Grey' Market in Antiquities." *Journal of Contemporary Criminal Justice* 24(3):225–42.

Boyer, Kate. (2010). "Of Care and Commodities: Breast Milk and the New Politics of Mobile Biosubstances." *Progress in Human Geography* 34(1):5–20.

Boyer, Kate and Maia Boswell-Penc. (2010). "Breast Pumps: A Feminist Technology, or (Yet) 'More Work for Mother'?" In Linda L. Layne, Sharra L. Vostral and Kate Boyer (eds) *Feminist Technology*. Chicago, IL: University of Illinois Press, pp. 119–35.

Brady, June Pauline. (2012). "Marketing Breast Milk Substitutes: Problems and Perils throughout the World." *Archives of Disease in Childhood* 97(6):529–32.

Breakey, Alicia A., Katie Hinde, Claudia R. Valeggia and Peter T. Ellison. (2015). "Illness in Breastfeeding Infants Relates to Concentration of Lactoferrin and Secretory Immunoglobulin A in Mother's Milk." *Evolution, Medicine, and Public Health* 1:21–31.

Brekke, Ole Andreas and Thorvald Sirnes. (2011). "Biosociality, Biocitizenship, and the New Regime of Hope and Despair: Interpreting 'Portraits of Hope' and the 'Mehmet Case'." *New Genetics and Society* 30(4):347–74.

Brookes, Alastair and Douglas M. Bowley. (2014). "Tongue Tie: The Evidence for Frenotomy." *Early Human Development* 90(11):765–8.

Bucholtz, Mary. (1996). "'Why Be Normal?': Language and Identity Practices in a Community of Nerd Girls." *Language in Society* 28(2):203–23.

Budzynska, Katarzyna, Zoe E. Gardner, Jean-Jacques Dugoua, Tieraona Low Dog and Paula Gardiner. (2012). "Systematic Review of Breastfeeding and Herbs." *Breastfeeding Medicine* 7(6):489–503.

Carroll, Katherine. (2014). "Body Dirt or Liquid Gold? How the 'Safety' of Donated Breastmilk Is Constructed for Use in Neonatal Intensive Care." *Social Studies of Science* 44(3):466–85.

Carroll, Katherine. (2015). "Breastmilk Donation as Care Work." In Tanya Cassidy and Abdullahi El Tom (eds) *Ethnographies of Breastfeeding: Cultural Contexts and Confrontations*. London: Bloomsbury Academic, pp. 173–86.

Carroll, Katherine and Kenneth R. Herrmann. (2013). "The Cost of Using Donor Human Milk in the NICU to Achieve Exclusively Human Milk Feeding through 32 Weeks Postmenstrual Age." *Breastfeeding Medicine* 8(3):286–90.

Carroll, Katherine and Brydan Lenne. (2019). "Suppress and Express: Breastmilk Donation after Neonatal Death." In Charlotte Beyer and Andrea Robertson (eds) *Mothers Without Their Children*. Bradford, Ontario: Demeter Press, pp. 229–44.

Carroll, Katherine E., Brydan S. Lenne, Kerri McEgan, Opie Gillian, Lisa H. Amir, Sandra Bredemeyer, Ben Hartmann, Rachel Jones, Pieter Koorts, Helen McConachy, Patricia Mumford and Jan Polverino. (2014). "Breast Milk Donation after Neonatal Death in Australia: A Report." *International Breastfeeding Journal* 9:23.

Carsten, Janet. (1995). "The Substance of Kinship and the Heat of the Hearth: Feeding, Personhood, and Relatedness among Malays in Pulau Langkawi." *American Ethnologist* 22(2):223–41.

Carter, Shannon K. (2010). "Beyond Control: Body and Self in Women's Childbearing Narratives." *Sociology of Health & Illness* 32(7):993–1009.

Carter, Shannon K. (2017). "Body-Led Mothering: Constructions of the Breast in Attachment Parenting Literature." *Women's Studies International Forum* 62:17–24.

Carter, Shannon K. and Beatriz M. Reyes-Foster. (2016). "Pure Gold for Broken Bodies: Discursive Techniques Constructing Milk Banking and Peer Milk Sharing in the US." *Symbolic Interaction* 39(3):353–73.

Carter, Shannon K. and Beatriz Reyes-Foster. (2017). "Peer Breast Milk Sharing as Resistance to Patriarchal Control." *Journal of Mother Studies* 2, https://jourms.wordpress.com/peer-breast-milk-sharing-as-resistance-to-patriarchal-control

Carter, Shannon K. and Beatriz M. Reyes-Foster. (2020). "Considering Materiality: The Utility of Actor-Network Theory to Study Social Problems." In J. Travino and A. Marvasti (eds) *Researching Social Problems*. New York, NY: Routledge, pp. 139–55.

Carter, Shannon K., Beatriz M. Reyes-Foster and J. Scott Carter. (2018). "'Breast Is Best, Donor Next': Peer Breastmilk Sharing in Contemporary Western Motherhood." *Sociological Inquiry* 88(4):673–95.

Carter, Shannon K., Beatriz Reyes-Foster and Tiffany L. Rogers. (2015). "Liquid Gold or Russian Roulette? Risk and Human Milk Sharing in the U.S. News Media." *Health, Risk & Society* 17(1):30–45.

Cassar-Uhl, Diana and Penny Liberatos. (2018). "Use of Shared Milk among Breastfeeding Mothers with Lactation Insufficiency." *Maternal & Child Nutrition* 14(S6):e12594.

Cassidy, Tanya. (2012a). "Making 'Milky Matches': Globalization, Maternal Trust and 'Lactivist' Online Networking." *Journal of the Motherhood Initiative for Research and Community Involvement* 3(1):226–40.

Cassidy, Tanya M. (2012b). "Mothers, Milk, and Money: Maternal Corporeal Generosity, Social Psychological Trust, and Value in Human Milk Exchange." *Journal of the Motherhood Initiative for Research and Community Involvement* 3(1): 96–111.

Cassidy, Tanya M. and Abdullahi El Tom. (2010). "Comparing Sharing and Banking Milk: Issues of Gift Exchange and Community in the Sudan and Ireland." In Rhonda Shaw and Alison Bartlett (eds) *Giving Breastmilk: Body Ethics and Contemporary Breastfeeding Practice*. Toronto: Demeter Press, pp. 110–21.

CDC. (2018). *Breastfeeding Report Card: United States, 2018*, Atlanta, GA: Centers for Disease Control and Prevention, www.cdc.gov/breastfeeding/pdf/2018breastfeedingreportcard.pdf

Charmaz, Kathy and Linda Liska Belgrave. (2012). "Qualitative Interviewing and Grounded Theory Analysis." In Jaber F. Gubrium, James A. Holstein, Amir B. Marvasti and Karyn D. McKinney (eds) *The Sage Handbook of Interview Research: The Complexity of the Craft*. Thousand Oaks, CA: Sage, pp. 347–65.

Clarke, Mike, Gerard Savage, Valerie Smith, Deirdre Daly, Declan Devane, Mechthild M. Gross, Susanne Grylka-Baeschlin, Patricia Healy, Sandra Morano, Jane Nicoletti and Cecily Begley. (2015). "Improving the Organisation of Maternal Health Service Delivery and Optimising Childbirth by Increasing Vaginal Birth after Caesarean Section through Enhanced Women-centred Care (OptiBIRTH trial): Study Protocol for a Randomised Controlled Trial (ISRCTN10612254)." *Trials* 16(1):542.

Comte, Auguste. (1974 [1855]). *The Positive Philosophy*. Harriet Martineau (trans.). New York, NY: AMS Press.

Coole, Diana and Samantha Frost. (2010). *New Materialisms: Ontology, Agency, and Politics*. Durham, NC: Duke University Press.

Côté, Isabel and Kévin Lavoie. (2019). "A Child Wanted by Two, Conceived by Several: Lesbian-parent Families Negotiating Procreation with a Known Donor." *Journal of GLBT Family Studies* 15(2): 165-185.

Cross-Barnet, Caitlin, Marycatherine Augustyn, Susan Gross, Amy Resnik and David Paige. (2012). "Long-Term Breastfeeding Support: Failing Mothers in Need." *Maternal and Child Health Journal* 16(9):1926–32.

Crossley, Michele L. (2009). "Breastfeeding as a Moral Imperative: An Autoethnographic Study." *Sage Journals Feminism & Psychology* 19(1):71–87.

Dalla Costa, Mariarosa and Selma James. (1972). *The Power of Women and the Subversion of the Community*. Bristol: Falling Wall Press.

David, Stephanie Dawson. (2011). "Legal Commentary on the Internet Sale of Human Milk." *Public Health Reports* 126(2):165–6.

de Alencar, Lucienne Christine Estevez and Eliane Maria Fleury Seidle. (2009). "Breast Milk Donation: Women's Donor Experience." *Rev Saude Publica* 43(1):70–7.

Durkheim, Emile. (1947 [1912]). *The Elementary Forms of Religious Life*. New York, NY: Free Press.

Dutton, Judy. (2011). "Liquid Gold: The Booming Market for Human Breast Milk." *Wired*, 17 May.

Eagle, Ryan Bowles. (2019). "'Have you Tried Ginger?': Severe Pregnancy Sickness and Intensive Mothering on Instagram." *Feminist Media Studies* 19(5):767–9.

Eats on Feets. (n.d.). "The Four Pillars of Safe Breast Milk Sharing." Eats on Feets, www.eatsonfeets.org/#fourPillars

Eglash, Anne, Liliana Simon and The Academy of Breastfeeding Medicine. (2017). "ABM Clinical Protocol #8: Human Milk Storage Information for Home Use for Full-Term Infants, Revised 2017." *Breastfeeding Medicine* 12(7):390–5.

Eidelman, Arthur I. (2015). "The Ultimate Social Network: Breastmilk Sharing via the Internet." *Breastfeeding Medicine* 10(5):231.

Emerson, Robert M. and Rachel I. Fretz. (2001). "Participant Observation." In Paul Atkinson, Amanda Coffey, Sara Delamont, John Lofland and Lyn Lofland (eds) *Handbook of Ethnography*. Los Angeles, CA: Sage, pp. 352–68.

Faircloth, Charlotte. (2013). *Militant Lactivism?: Attachment Parenting and Intensive Motherhood in the UK and France*. Oxford: Berghahn Books.

Falls, Susan. (2017). *White Gold: Stories of Breast Milk Sharing*. Lincoln, NE: University of Nebraska Press.

Fentiman, Linda. (2009). "Marketing Mothers' Milk: The Commodification of Breastfeeding and the New Markets for Breast Milk and Infant Formula." *Nevada Law Journal* 10:29–81.

Fildes, Valerie. (1987). *Breasts, Bottles, and Babies: A History of Infant Feeding*. Edinburgh: Edinburgh University Press.

Fomaro, Matthew. (2003). "A Parallel Problem: Grey Market Goods and the Internet." *Journal of Technology Law & Policy* 8:69.

Foss, Katherine A. (2017). *Breastfeeding and Media: Exploring Conflicting Discourses that Threaten Public Health*. Cham: Palgrave Macmillan.

Foucault, Michel. (1978). *The History of Sexuality, Volume I: An Introduction*. New York, NY: Pantheon Books.

Foucault, Michel. (2003). *"Society Must Be Defended": Lectures at the Collège De France, 1975–1976*. New York, NY: Picador.

Fox, Renée and Judith Swazey. (1992). *Spare Parts: Organ Replacement in American Society*. Oxford: Oxford University Press.

Free, Cathy. (2019). "Why These Bikers Crisscross New York Delivering Donated Breast Milk." *The Washington Post*, 4 November.

Friedan, Betty. (1963[2001]). *The Feminine Mystique*. New York, NY: W.W. Norton & Company.

Fuchs, Christian. (2017). *Social Media: A Critical Introduction*. Thousand Oaks, CA: Sage.

Gaard, Greta. (2013). "Toward a Feminist Postcolonial Milk Studies." *American Quarterly* 65(3):595–618.

Geraghty, Sheela R., Julie E. Heier and Kathleen M. Rasmussen. (2011). "Got Milk? Sharing Human Milk via the Internet." *Public Health Reports* 126(2):161–4.

Geraghty, Sheela R., Kelly A. McNamara, Chelsea E. Dillon, Joseph S. Hogan, Jesse J. Kwiek and Sarah A. Keim. (2013). "Buying Human Milk via the Internet: Just a Click Away." *Breastfeeding Medicine* 8(6):474–8.

Geraghty, Sheela R., Kelly McNamara, Jesse J. Kwiek, Lynette Rogers, Mark A. Klebanoff, Molly Augustine and Sarah A. Keim. (2015). "Tobacco Metabolites and Caffeine in Human Milk Purchased via the Internet." *Breastfeeding Medicine* 10(9):419–24.

Giles, Fiona. (2003). *Fresh Milk: The Secret Life of Breasts*. Crows Nest: Allen and Unwin.

Giles, Fiona. (2010). "From 'Gift of Loss' to Self-Care: The Significance of Induced Lactation in Takashi Miike's Visitor Q." In Rhonda Shaw and Alison Bartlett (eds) *Giving Breastmilk: Body Ethics and Contemporary Breastfeeding Practice*. Ontario, Canada: Demeter Press, pp. 236–49.

Giles, Fiona. (2017). "Towards Social Maternity: *Where's the Mother? Stories from a Transgender Dad* as a Case Study of Human Milk Sharing." In Rhonda M. Shaw (eds) *Bioethics Beyond Altruism: Donating and Transforming Human Biological Materials.* Cham: Palgrave MacMillan, pp. 291–318.

Golden, Janet. (1996). *A Social History of Wet Nursing in America: From Breast to Bottle.* Cambridge: Cambridge University Press.

Goodman, David. (2001). "Ontology Matters: The Relational Materiality of Nature and Agro-Food Studies." *Sociologia Ruralis* 41(2):182–200.

Granju, Katie Allison and Betsy Kennedy. (1999). *Attachment Parenting: Instinctive Care for your Baby and Young Child.* New York, NY: Simon and Schuster.

Gribble, Karleen D. (2012). "Biomedical Ethics and Peer-to-Peer Milk Sharing." *Clinical Lactation* 3(3):108–111.

Gribble, Karleen D. (2013). "Peer-to-Peer Milk Donors' and Recipients' Experiences and Perceptions of Donor Milk Banks." *Journal of Obstetric, Gynecologic & Neonatal Nursing* 42(4):451–61.

Gribble, Karleen D. (2014a). "Perception and Management of Risk in Internet-Based Peer-to-Peer Milk Sharing." *Early Child Development and Care* 184(1):84–98.

Gribble, Karleen D. (2014b). " 'I'm Happy to Be Able to Help': Why Women Donate Milk to a Peer Via Internet-Based Milk Sharing Networks." *Breastfeeding Medicine* 9(5):251–6.

Gribble, Karleen D. (2014c). " 'A Better Alternative': Why Women Use Peer-to-Peer Shared Milk." *Breastfeeding Review* 22(1):11–21.

Gribble, Karleen. (2018). " 'Someone's Generosity has Formed a Bond Between Us': Interpersonal Relationships in Internet-Facilitated Peer-to-Peer Milk Sharing." *Maternal & Child Nutrition* 14:e12575.

Gribble, Karleen D. and Bernice L. Hausman. (2012). "Milk Sharing and Formula Feeding: Infant Feeding Risks in Comparative Perspective?" *The Australian Medical Journal* 5(5):275.

Halse, Christine. (2009). "Bio-citizenship: Virtue Discourses and the Birth of the Bio-citizen." In Jan Wright and Valerie Harwood (eds) *Biopolitics and the "Obesity Epidemic."* New York, NY: Routledge, pp. 53–67.

Han, Sallie. (2013). *Pregnancy in Practice: Expectation and Experience in the Contemporary US.* New York, NY: Berghahn Books.

Harrison, Laura. (2016). *Brown Bodies, White Babies: The Politics of Cross-Racial Surrogacy.* New York, NY: New York University Press.

Harrison, Laura. (2019). "Milk Money: Race, Gender, and Breast Milk 'Donation'." *Signs: Journal of Women in Culture and Society* 44(2):281–306.

Hartmann, Heidi. (1976). "Capitalism, Patriarchy, and Job Segregation by Sex." *Signs: Journal of Women and Culture in Society* 1(3):137–69.

Hassan, Narin. (2010). "Milk Markets: Technology, the Lactating Body, and New Forms of Consumption." *Women's Studies Quarterly* 39(3/4):209–28.

Hausman, Bernice L. (2007). "Things (Not) to do with Breasts in Public: Maternal Embodiment and the Biocultural Politics of Infant Feeding." *New Literary History* 38(3): 479–504.

Hausman, Bernice L. (2014). *Mother's Milk: Breastfeeding Controversies in American Culture.* New York, NY: Routledge.

Hays, Sharon. (1996). *The Cultural Contradictions of Motherhood.* New Haven, CT: Yale University Press.

HealthDay News. (2019). "AAP: Most Moms Unconcerned with Informal Milk Sharing." *Physician's Weekly*, 24 October.

Hermann, Kenneth and Katherine Carroll. (2014). "An Exclusively Human Milk Diet Reduces Necrotizing Enterocolitis." *Breastfeeding Medicine* 9(4):184–90.

Hewlett, Barry S. and Steve Winn. (2014). "Allomaternal nursing in humans." *Current Anthropology* 55(2):200–29.

Hinde, Katie. (2016). "Breast Milk & Baby Spit." *Mammals Suck… Milk!* [Blog] 29 January, http://mammalssuck.blogspot.com/2016/01/breast-milk-baby-spit.html

Hinde, Katie and Lauren Milligan. (2011). "Primate Milk: Proximate Mechanisms and Ultimate Perspectives." *Evolutionary Anthropology* 20:9–23.

Hochschild, Arlie Russell. (1983). *The Managed Heart: Commercialization of Human Feeling.* Berkeley, CA: University of California Press.

Hochschild, Arlie Russell. (1989). *The Second Shift: Working Parents and the Revolution at Home.* New York, NY: Viking.

Hookway, Nicholas, Shandell Elmer and Mai Frandsen. (2017). "Risk, Morality and Emotion: Social Media Responses to Pregnant Women who Smoke." *Health, Risk & Society* 19(5–6):246–59.

HMBANAa (Human Milk Banking Association of North America). (n.d.). "Locations." HMBANA, www.hmbana.org/locations.

HMBANAb. (n.d.). "Donor Human Milk: Ensuring Safety and Ethical Allocation." HMBANA.

Hovav, April. (2019). "Producing Moral Palatability in the Mexican Surrogacy Market." *Gender & Society* 33(2):273–295.

Jansson, Maria. (2009). "Feeding Children and Protecting Women: The Emergence of Breastfeeding as an International Concern." *Women's Studies International Forum* 32(3):240–8.

Johnson, Christopher M. (2001). "A Survey of Current Research on Online Communities of Practice." *The Internet and Higher Education* 4(1):45–60.

Johnson, Katherine M. (2019). "Making Milk and Money: Contemporary Mothers' Orientations to Breastfeeding and Work." *Sociological Forum* 34(4):883–903.

Johnson, Katherine M. and Colleen Salpini. (2017). "Working and Nursing: Navigating Job and Breastfeeding Demands at Work." *Community, Work & Family* 20(4):479–96.

Johnson, Sophia Alice. (2014). "'Maternal Devices', Social Media and the Self-Management of Pregnancy, Mothering and Child Health." *Societies* 4(2):330–50.

Jones, Frances. (2013). "Milk Sharing: How it Undermines Breastfeeding." *Breastfeeding Review* 21(3):21.

Kehily, Mary Jane and Lydia Martens. (2014). "For the Love of Small Things: Consumerism and the Making of Maternal Identities." *Young Consumers* 15(3):227–38.

Keim, Sarah A., Joseph S. Hogan, Kelly A. McNamara, Vishnu Gudimetla, Chelsea E. Dillon, Jesse J. Kwiek and Sheela R. Geraghty. (2013). "Microbial Contamination of Human Milk Purchased Via the Internet." *Pediatrics* 132(5):e1227–e35.

Keim, Sarah A., Manjusha M. Kulkarni, Kelly A. McNamara, Sheela R. Geraghty, Rachael M. Billock, Rachel Ronau, Joseph S. Hogan and Jesse J. Kwiek. (2015). "Cow's Milk Contamination of Human Milk Purchased Via the Internet." *Pediatrics* 135(5):1–6.

Kelleher, Christa M. (2006). "The Physical Challenges of Early Breastfeeding." *Social Science & Medicine* 63(10):2727–38.

Kertzer, David. (1999). "Syphilis, Foundlings, and Wetnurses in Nineteenth Century Italy." *Journal of Social History* 32(3):589–602.

Kim, Jae H. and Elizabeth B. Froh. (2012). "What Nurses Need to Know Regarding Nutritional and Immunobiological Properties of Human Milk." *Journal of Obstetric, Gynecologic & Neonatal Nursing* 41:122–37.

Knaak, Stephanie J. (2006). "The Problem with Breastfeeding Discourse." *Canadian Journal of Public Health* 97(5):412–14.

Knaak, Stephanie J. (2010). "Contextualizing Risk, Constructing Choice: Breastfeeding and Good Mothering in Risk Society." *Health, Risk & Society* 12(4):345–55.

Kotlow, Lawrence A. (2013). "Diagnosing and Understanding the Maxillary Lip-Tie (Superior Labial, the Maxillary Labial Frenum) as it Relates to Breastfeeding." *Journal of Human Lactation* 29(4):458–64.

Kroløkke, Charlotte and Michael Nebeling Petersen. (2017). "Keeping it in the Family: Debating the Bio-intimacy of Uterine Transplants and Commercial Surrogacy." In Rhonda M. Shaw (ed) *Bioethics Beyond Altruism: Donating and Transforming Human Biological Materials*. Cham: Palgrave Macmillan, pp. 189–214.

Kukla, Rebecca. (2006). "Ethics and Ideology in Breastfeeding Advocacy Campaigns." *Hypatia* 21(1):157–80.

Landers, Susan and Ben T. Hartmann. (2013). "Donor Human Milk Banking and the Emergence of Milk Sharing." *Pediatric Clinics* 60(1):247–60.

Latour, Bruno. (2005). *Reassembling the Social: An Introduction to Actor-Network Theory*. New York, NY: Oxford University Press.

Lave, Jean. (1991). "Situated Learning in Communities of Practice." *Perspectives on Socially Shared Cognition* 2:63–82.

Lave, Jean and Etienne Wenger. (1991). *Situated Learning*. Cambridge: Cambridge University Press.

Law, John. (2009). "Actor Network Theory and Material Semiotics." in Bryan S. Turner (ed) *The New Blackwell Companion to Social Theory*. Chichester: Blackwell Publishing, pp. 141–58.

Law, Jules. (2000). "The Politics of Breastfeeding: Assessing Risk, Dividing Labor." *Signs* 25(2).

Lee, Ellie (2007). "Health, Morality, and Infant Feeding: British Mothers' Experiences of Formula Milk Use in the Early Weeks." *Sociology of Health and Illness* 29(7):1075–90.

Lee, Ellie. (2011). "Breast-Feeding Advocacy, Risk Society and Health Moralism: A Decade's Scholarship." *Sociology Compass* 5(12):1058–69.

Lee, Ellie J. (2008). "Living with Risk in the Age of "Intensive Motherhood": Maternal Identity and Infant Feeding." *Health, Risk & Society* 10(5):467–77.

Lee, Robyn. (2018a). *The Ethics and Politics of Breastfeeding: Power, Pleasure, Poetics*. Toronto: University of Toronto Press.

Lee, Robyn. (2018b). "Breastfeeding Bodies: Intimacies at Work." *Gender, Work & Organization* 25(1):77–90.

Lee, Robyn. (2019). "Commodifying Compassion: Affective Economies of Human Milk Exchange." *International Journal of Feminist Approaches to Bioethics* 12(2):92–116.

Lieber, Chavie. (2014). "Meet the Men who Drink Breast Milk." *The Cut*, 28 May.

Locatelli, Elisabetta. (2017). "Images of Breastfeeding on Instagram: Self-Representation, Publicness, and Privacy Management." *Social Media + Society* 3(2):1–14.

Locke, Abigail. (2009). "Natural versus Taught' Competing Discourses in Antenatal Breastfeeding Workshops." *Journal of Health Psychology* 14(3):435–46.

Locke, Abigail. (2018). "Parenting Ideologies, Infant Feeding and Popular Culture." In Sally Dowling, David Pontin and Kate Boyer (eds) *Social Experiences of Breastfeeding: Building Bridges between Research, Policy and Practice*. Bristol: Policy Press, pp. 147–61.

Long, Debbi. (2003). "Breast Sharing: Cross-Feeding among Australian Women." *Health Sociology Review* 12(2):103–10.

Longhurst, Robyn. (2001). *Bodies: Exploring Fluid Boundaries*. London: Routledge.

Lönnerdal, Bo. (2013). "Bioactive Proteins in Breast Milk." *Journal of Paediatrics and Child Health* 49(Supp. 1):1–7.

Lozoff, Betsy. (1983). "Birth and 'Bonding' in Non-Industrial Societies." *Developmental Medicine & Child Neurology* 25(5):595–600.

Lupton, Deborah. (2013). "Infant embodiment and interembodiment: A review of sociocultural perspectives." *Childhood* 20(1): 37–50.

Lupton, Deborah, Sarah Pedersen and Gareth M. Thomas. (2016). "Parenting and Digital Media: From the Early Web to Contemporary Digital Society." *Sociology Compass* 10(8):730–43.

Macdonald, Margaret. (2006). "Gender Expectations: Natural Bodies and Natural Births in the New Midwifery in Canada." *Medical Anthropology Quarterly* 20(2):235–56.

MacDonald, Trevor, Joy Noel-Weiss, Diana West, Michelle Walks, MaryLynne Biener, Alanna Kibbe and Elizabeth Myler. (2016). "Transmasculine Individuals' Experiences with Lactation, Chestfeeding, and Gender Identity: A Qualitative Study." *BMC Pregnancy and Childbirth* 16:106.

MacDorman, Marian F., and Eugene Declercq. (2019). "Trends and State Variations in Out-of-hospital Births in the United States, 2004–2017." *Birth* 46(2): 279–288.

Mackendrick, Norah. (2014). "More Work for Mother: Chemical Body Burdens as a Maternal Responsibility." *Gender & Society* 28(5):705–28.

Malacrida, Claudia and Tiffany Boulton. (2012). "Women's Perceptions of Childbirth 'Choices': Competing Discourses of Motherhood, Sexuality, and Selflessness." *Gender & Society* 26(5):748–72.

Mamo, Laura. (2007). *Queering Reproduction: Achieving Pregnancy in the Age of Technoscience*. Durham, NC: Duke University Press.

Marshall, Joyce L., Mary Godfrey and Mary J. Renfrew. (2007). "Being a 'Good Mother': Managing Breastfeeding and Merging Identities." *Social Science & Medicine* 65(10):2147–59.

Marx, Karl. (1967 [1867]). *Capital, Volume 1: A Critical Analysis of Capitalist Production.* International Publishers.

Mathews, Joan and Kathleen Zadak. (1991). "The Alternative Birth Movement in the United States: History and Current Status." *Women and Health* 17(1):39–56.

Mauss, Marcel. (1950 [1925]). *The Gift: The Form and Reason for Exchange in Archaic Societies.* W.D. Halls (trans.). New York, NY: Norton.

McCloskey, Rebecca J. and Sharvari Karandikar. (2019). "Peer-to-Peer Human Milk Sharing: Recipient Mothers' Motivations, Stress, and Postpartum Mental Health." *Breastfeeding Medicine* 14(2):88–97.

Medolac. (2018). "Medolac: A Public Benefit Corporation." Medolac, www.medolac.com

Meins, Alexa R., Ardith Z. Doorenbos, Linda Eaton, Debra Gordon, Brian Theodore and David Tauben. (2015). "TelePain: A Community of Practice for Pain Management." *Journal of Pain & Relief* 4(2):177.

Miller, Elizabeth. (2015). "Milk Immunity and Reproductive Status among Ariaal Women of Northern Kenya." *Annals of Human Biology* 42(1):76–83.

Nelson, Roxanne. (2012). "Breast Milk Sharing is Making a Comeback, But Should It?" *American Journal of Nursing* 112(6):19–20.

Novas, Carlos. (2006). "The Political Economy of Hope: Patients Organizations, Science and Biovalue. " *BioSocieties* 1(3):289–305.

Oakley, Ann. (1974[2019]). *The Sociology of Housework.* Bristol, UK: Policy Press.

Oakley, Ann. (2018). *From Here to Maternity: Becoming a Mother (reissue).* Bristol, UK: Policy Press.

O'Donohoe, Stephanie, Margaret Hogg, Pauline Maclaran, Lydia Martens and Lorna Stevens. (2013). *Motherhoods, Markets and Consumption: The Making of Mothers in Contemporary Western Cultures.* New York, NY: Routledge.

Onat, Güliz, and Hediye Karakoç. (2019). "Informal Breast Milk Sharing in a Muslim Country: The Frequency, Practice, Risk Perception, and Risk Reduction Strategies Used by Mothers." *Breastfeeding Medicine* 14(8):597–602.

Oreg, Alylet. (2019). "Milk Donation after Losing One's Baby: Adopting a Donor Identity as a Means of Coping with Loss." *Social Science & Medicine* 238:112519.

Osbaldiston, Richard and Leigh A. Mingle. (2007). "Characterization of Human Milk Donors." *Journal of Human Lactation* 23(4):350–57.

O'Sullivan, Elizabeth J., Sheela R. Geraghty and Kathleen M. Rasmussen. (2018). "Awareness and Prevalence of Human Milk Sharing and Selling in the United States." *Maternal & Child* Nutrition 14(S6):e12567.

Owens, Nicole, Shannon K. Carter, Chelsea J. Nordham and Jason A. Ford. (2018). "Neutralizing the Maternal Breast: Accounts of Public Breastfeeding by African American Mothers." *Journal of Family Issues* 39(2):430–50.

Palmquist, Aunchalee E.L. (2015). "Demedicalizing Breastmilk: The Discourses, Practices, and Identities of Informal Milk Sharing." In Tanya Cassidy and Abdullahi El Tom (eds) *Ethnographies of Breastfeeding: Cultural Contexts and Confrontations*. London: Bloomsbury Academic, pp. 23–44.

Palmquist, Aunchalee and Kirsten Doehler. (2014). "Contextualizing Online Human Milk Sharing: Structural Factors and Lactation Disparity among Middle Income Women in the U.S." *Social Science & Medicine* 122:140–7.

Palmquist, Aunchalee E. L. and Kirsten Doehler. (2016). "Human Milk Sharing Practices in the U.S.". *Maternal & Child Nutrition* 12(2):278–90.

Palmquist, Aunchalee E. L., Maryanne T. Perrin, Diana Cassar-Uhl, Karleen D. Gribble, Angela B. Bond, and Tanya Cassidy. (2019). "Current trends in research on human milk exchange for infant feeding." *Journal of Human Lactation* 35(3): 453–477.

Parkes, Peter. (2001). "Alternative Social Structures and Foster Relations in the Hindu Kush: Milk Kinship Allegiance in Former Mountain Kingdoms of Northern Pakistan." *Comparative Studies in Society and History* 43(1):4–36.

Parkes, Peter. (2004). "Milk Kinship in Southeast Europe: Alternative Social Structures and Foster Relations in the Caucasus and the Balkans." *Social Anthropology* 12(3):341–58.

Patel, Aloka and Jae Kim. (2018). "Human Milk and Necrotizing Enterocolitis." *Seminars in Pediatric Surgery* 27(1):34–8.

Paynter, Martha Jane and Lisa Goldberg. (2018). "A Critical Review of Human Milk Sharing Using an Intersectional Feminist Framework: Implications for Practice." *Midwifery* 66:141–7.

Pedersen, Sarah. (2016). "The Good, the Bad and the 'Good Enough' Mother on the UK Parenting Forum Mumsnet." *Women's Studies International Forum* 59:32–8.

Perrin, Andrew and Monica Anderson. (2019). "Share of U.S. Adults Using Social Media, Including Facebook, is Mostly Unchanged Since 2018." Pew Research Center, www.pewresearch.org/fact-tank/2019/04/10/share-of-u-s-adults-using-social-media-including-facebook-is-mostly-unchanged-since-2018

Perrin, Maryanne Tigchelaar, L. Suzanne Goodell, Jonathan C. Allen and April Fogleman. (2014). "A Mixed-Methods Observational Study of Human Milk Sharing Communities on Facebook." *Breastfeeding Medicine* 9(3):128–34.

Perrin, Maryanne Tigchelaar, L. Suzanne Goodell, April Fogleman, Hannah Pettus, Amanda L. Bodenheimer and Aunchalee E. L. Palmquist. (2016). "Expanding the Supply of Pasteurized Donor Milk: Understanding Why Peer-to-Peer Milk Sharers in the United States Do Not Donate to Milk Banks." *Journal of Human Lactation* 32(2):229–37.

Perrin, Maryanne T., April D. Fogleman, Destiny D. Davis, Courtney H. Wimer, Kenneth G. Vogel and Aunchalee E. L. Palmquist. (2018). "A Pilot Study on Nutrients, Antimicrobial Proteins, and Bacteria in Commerce-Free Models for Exchanging Expressed Human Milk in the USA." *Maternal & Child Nutrition* 14:e12566.

Peters, Michael A. and Priya Venkatesan. (2010). "Biocapitalism and the Politics of Life." *Geopolitics, History, and International Relations* 2(2):100–22.

Plummer, Ken. (1993). *Intimate Citizenship: Private Decisions and Public Dialogues*. Seattle, WA: University of Washington Press.

Porter, Jennifer. (2018). "Choreographing Pumping: Remaking the 'Ideal' Worker through Maternal Embodiment in the Workplace." *Social & Cultural Geography* 19(4):520–41.

Porter, Maree, Ian H. Kerridge and Christopher F. C. Jordens. (2012). "'Good Mothering' or 'Good Citizenship'?" *Journal of Bioethical Inquiry* 9(1):41–7.

Prolacta. (2018). "Prolacta Bioscience: Advancing the Science of Human Milk." Prolacta, www.prolacta.com

Quinn, E. A. (2018). "Milk, Medium Chain Fatty Acids and Human Evolution." In Cecilia Tomori, Aunchalee E. L. Palmquist and E. A. Quinn (eds) *Breastfeeding: New Anthropological Approaches*. New York, NY: Routledge, pp. 112–26.

Quinn, Elizabeth, Kesang Diki Bista and Geoff Childs. (2016). "Milk at Altitude: Human Milk Macronutrient Composition in a High-Altitude Adapted Population of Tibetans." *American Journal of Physical Anthropology* 159:233–43.

Quinn, Elizabeth, F. E. Largado, Michael Power and Christopher Kuzawa. (2012). "Predictors of Breast Milk Macronutrient Composition in Filipino Mothers." *American Journal of Human Biology* 24:433–540.

Rabinow, Paul. (1996). "Artificiality and Enlightenment: From Sociobiology to Biosociality." In *Essays on the Anthropology of Reason*. Princeton, NJ: Princeton University Press, pp. 234–52.

Ramli, Noraida and Nor Roshidah Ibrahim. (2010). "Human Milk Banks: The Benefits and Issues in an Islamic Setting." *Eastern Journal of Medicine* 15(4):163.

Ranmuthugala, Geetha, Jennifer J. Plumb, Frances C. Cunningham, Andrew Georgiou, Johanna I. Westbrook and Jeffrey Braithwaite. (2011). "How and Why are Communities of Practice Established in the Healthcare Sector? A Systematic Review of the Literature." *BMC Health Services Research* 11(1):273.

Reich, Jennifer A. (2016). *Calling the Shots: Why Parents Reject Vaccines*. New York, NY: New York University Press.

Reyes-Foster, Beatriz M. and Shannon K. Carter. (2018a). "Suspect Bodies, Suspect Milk: Milk Sharing, Wetnursing, and the Specter of Syphilis in the Twenty-First Century." In K. Nixon and L. Servitje (eds) *Syphilis and Subjectivity: From the Victorians to the Present*. Cham: Palgrave Macmillan, pp. 91-112.

Reyes-Foster, Beatriz M. and Shannon K. Carter. (2018b). "Mothers, Milk and Morals: Peer Milk Sharing as Moral Motherwork in Central Florida." In C. Tomori, A. E. L. Palmquist and E. A. Quinn (eds) *Breastfeeding: New Anthropological Approaches*. New York, NY: Routledge, pp. 97–111.

Reyes-Foster, Beatriz M. and Shannon K. Carter. (2018c). " 'That's Not the Milk Sharing I'm Doing': Responses to a Pediatrics Article from Women Who Milk Share." *Human Organization* 77(3):262–72.

Reyes-Foster, Beatriz M., Shannon K. Carter and Melanie Sberna Hinojosa. (2015). "Milk Sharing in Practice: A Descriptive Analysis of Peer Breastmilk Sharing." *Breastfeeding Medicine* 10(5):263–9.

Reyes-Foster, Beatriz, Shannon K. Carter and Melanie Sberna Hinojosa. (2017). "Human Milk Handling and Storage Practices among Peer Milk-Sharing Mothers." *Journal of Human Lactation* 33(1):173–80.

Rippeyoung, Phyllis L.F. (2009). "Feeding the State: Breastfeeding and Women's Well-Being in Context." *Journal of the Motherhood Initiative for Research and Community Involvement* 11(1):36–48.

Rose, Nikolas. (1996). *Inventing Our Selves: Psychology, Power, and Personhood*. Cambridge: Cambridge University Press.

Rose, Nikolas and Carlos Novas. (2005). "Biological Citizenship." In Aihwa Ong and Stephen J. Collier (eds) *Global Assemblages: Technology, Politics, and Ethics as Anthropological Problems*. Malden, MA: Blackwell Publishing, pp. 439–63.

Rosenberg, Kenneth, Carissa Eastham, Laurin Kasehagen and Alfredo Sandoval. (2008). "Marketing Infant Formula Through Hospitals: The Impact of Commercial Hospital Discharge Packs on Breastfeeding." *American Journal of Public Health* 98(2):290–5.

Rudrappa, Sharmila and Caitlyn Collins. (2015). "Altruistic Agencies and Compassionate Consumers: Moral Framing of Transnational Surrogacy." *Gender & Society* 29(6):937–59.

Ryan, Kath, Paul Bissel and Jo Alexander. (2010). "Moral Work in Women's Narratives of Breastfeeding." *Social Science & Medicine* 70:951–8.

Ryan, Kath, Victoria Team and Jo Alexander. (2017). "The Theory of Agency and Breastfeeding." *Psychology & Health* 32(3):312–29.

Ryan, Kath, Victoria Team and Jo Alexander. (2013). "Expressionists of the Twenty-First Century: The Commodification and Commercialization of Expressed Breast Milk." *Medical Anthropology* 32(5):467–86.

Ryan, Kath, Les Todres and Jo Alexander. (2011). "Calling, Permission and Fulfillment: The Interembodied Experience of Breastfeeding." *Qualitative Health Research* 21(6):731–42.

Schmied, Virginia and Lesley Barclay. (1999). "Connection and Pleasure, Disruption and Distress: Women's Experience of Breastfeeding." *Journal of Human Lactation* 15(4):325–34.

Schmied, Virginia and Deborah Lupton. (2001). "Blurring the Boundaries: Breastfeeding and Maternal Subjectivity." *Sociology of Health & Illness* 23(2):234–50.

Schafer, Ellen J., Sato Ashida and Aunchalee E. L. Palmquist. (2018). "Psychosocial Dimensions of Human Milk Sharing." *Maternal & Child Nutrition* 14:e12606.

Sears, William and Martha Sears. (2001). *The Attachment Parenting Book: A Commonsense Guide to Understanding and Nurturing your Baby*. New York, NY: Little, Brown and Company.

Shaikh, Ulfat and Omar Ahmed. (2006). "Islam and Infant Feeding." *Breastfeeding Medicine* 1(3):164–67.

Shaw, Rhonda. (2004a). "The Virtues of Cross-Nursing and the 'Yuk Factor'." *Australian Feminist Studies* 19(45):287–99.

Shaw, Rhonda. (2004b). "Performing Breastfeeding: Embodiment, Ethics and the Maternal Subject." *Feminist Review* 78(1):99–116.

Shaw, Rhonda M. (2007). "Cross-Nursing, Ethics and Giving Breast Milk in the Contemporary Context." *Women's Studies International Forum* 30:439–50.

Shaw, Rhonda. (2010). "Perspective on Ethics and Human Milk Banking." In Rhonda Shaw and Alison Bartlett (eds) *Giving Breastmilk: Body Ethics and Contemporary Breastfeeding*. Toronto: Demeter Press, pp. 83–97.

Shaw, Rhona M. (2015). *Ethics, Moral Life and the Body: Sociological Perspectives*. New York, NY: Palgrave.

Shaw, Rhonda M. (2017). "Bioethics beyond altruism." In Rhonda M. Shaw (ed) *Bioethics Beyond Altruism*. Cham: Palgrave Macmillan, pp. 3–31.

Shaw, Rhonda M. (2019). "Altruism, Solidarity and Affect in Live Kidney Donation and Breastmilk Sharing." *Sociology of Health & Illness* 41(3):553–66.

Shaw, Rhonda M. and Maggie Morgan. (2017). "Bio-Intimate Economies of Breastmilk Exchange: Peer-Milk Sharing and Donor Breastmilk in the NICU." In R. M. Shaw (ed) *Bioethics Beyond Altruism: Donating and Transforming Human Biological Materials*. Cham: Palgrave Macmillan, pp. 319–342.

Sherwood, Joan. (1995). "Treating Syphilis: The Wetnurse as Technology in an 18th Century Parisian Hospital." *Journal of the History of Medicine and Allied Sciences* 50(3):315–39.

Shildrick, Margrit. (2015). *Leaky Bodies and Boundaries: Feminism, Postmodernism and (Bio)Ethics*. London: Routledge.

Sim, Tin Fei, H. Laetitia Hattingh, Jillian Sherriff and Lisa B. G. Tee. (2015). "The Use, Perceived Effectiveness and Safety of Herbal Galactagogues during Breastfeeding: A Qualitative Study." *International Journal of Environmental Research and Public Health* 12(9):11050–71.

Simonds, Wendy, Barbara Katz Rothman and Bari Meltzer Norman. (2007). *Laboring On: Birth in Transition in the United States*. New York, NY: Routledge.

Singer, Peter. (2015). *The Most Good You Can Do: How Effective Altruism is Changing Ideas about Living Ethically*. Melbourne: Text Publishing.

Smyth, Lisa. (2008). "Gendered Spaces and Intimate Citizenship: The Case of Breastfeeding." *European Journal of Women's Studies* 15(2):83–99.

Soden, Rebecca, and John Halliday. (2000). "Rethinking vocational education: a case study in care." *International Journal of Lifelong Education* 19(2): 172–182.

Song, Felicia Wu, Jennifer Ellis West, Lisa Lundy and Nicole Smith Dahmen. (2012). "Women, Pregnancy, and Health Information Online: The Making of Informed Patients and Ideal Mothers." *Gender & Society* 26(5):773–98.

Sriraman, Natasha K., Amy E. Evans, Robert Lawrence, Lawrence Noble and Academy of Breastfeeding Medicine's Board of Directors. (2018). "Academy of Breastfeeding Medicine's 2017 Position Statement on Informal Breast Milk Sharing for the Term Healthy Infant." *Breastfeeding Medicine* 13(1).

Statista. (2020). "Number of Monthly Active Facebook Users Worldwide as of 4th Quarter 2019." Statista, www.statista.com/statistics/264810/number-of-monthly-active-facebook-users-worldwide

Stearns, Cindy A. (1999). "Breastfeeding and the Good Maternal Body." *Gender & Society* 13(3):308–25.

Stearns, Cindy A. (2009). "The Work of Breastfeeding." *Women's Studies Quarterly* 37(3 & 4):63–80.

Stearns, Cindy A. (2010). "The Breast Pump." In Rhonda Shaw and Alison Bartlett (eds) *Giving Breastmilk: Body Ethics and Contemporary Breastfeeding Practice.* Toronto: Demeter Press, pp. 11–23.

Stearns, Cindy A. (2013). "The Embodied Practices of Breastfeeding: Implications for Research and Policy." *Journal of Women, Politics & Policy* 34(4):359–70.

Steele, Sarah, Jeanine Martyn and Jens Foell. (2015). "Risks of the Unregulated Market in Human Breast Milk." *British Medical Journal* 350:h1485.

Strathern, Marilyn. (1990). *The Gender of the Gift: Problems with Women and Problems with Society in Melanesia.* Berkeley, CA: University of California Press.

Stuebe, Alison M., Karleen D. Gribble and A. E. Palmquist. (2014). "Differences between Online Milk Sales and Peer-to-Peer Milk Sharing." *Pediatrics* 132(5).

Struminger, Bruce, Sanjeev Arora, Sarah Zalud-Cerrato, David Lowrance and Tedd Ellerbrock. (2017). "Building Virtual Communities of Practice for Health." *The Lancet* 390(10095):632–4.

Sussman, George. (1982). *Selling Mother's Milk: The Wetnursing Business in France, 1715–1914.* Chicago, IL: University of Chicago Press.

Swanson, Kara. (2011). "Body Banks: A History of Milk Banks, Blood Banks, and Sperm Banks in the United States." *Enterprise & Society* 12(4):749–60.

Swanson, Kara. (2014). *Banking on the Body: The Market in Blood, Milk, and Sperm in Modern America.* Cambridge, MA: Harvard University Press.

Taylor, Erin N. and Lora Ebert Wallace. (2012). "For Shame: Feminism, Breastfeeding Advocacy, and Maternal Guilt." *Hypatia* 27(1):76–98.

Team, Victoria and Kath Ryan. (2014). "Expressed Breast Milk as Commodity: Disembodied Motherhood and Involved Fatherhood." In M. Nash (ed) *Reframing Reproduction: Conceiving Gendered Experiences, Genders and Sexualities in the Social Sciences*. London: Palgrave Macmillan, pp. 221–35.

Thomas, Gareth M., Deborah Lupton and Sarah Pedersen. (2018). "'The Appy for a Happy Pappy': Expectant Fatherhood and Pregnancy Apps." *Journal of Gender Studies* 27(7):759–70.

Thorley, Virginia. (2008). "Sharing Breast Milk: Wet-Nursing, Cross-Feeding, and Milk Donations." *Breastfeeding Review* 16(1):35–29.

Thorley, Virginia. (2009). "Mothers' Experience of Sharing Breastfeeding or Breastmilk: Co-Feeding in Australia, 1978–2008." *Breastfeeding Review* 17(1):9–18.

Thorley, Virginia. (2012). "Mothers' Experiences of Sharing Breastfeeding or Breastmilk, Part 2: The Early 21st Century." *Nursing Reports* 2(e2):4–12.

Thorley, Virginia. (2014). "Milk Siblingship, Religious and Secular: History, Applications, and Implications for Practice." *Women and Birth* 27(4):e16–e19.

Tiidenberg, Katrin and Nancy K. Baym. (2017). "Learn it, Buy it, Work it: Intensive Pregnancy on Instagram." *Social Media + Society* 3(1):1–13.

Titmuss, Richard M. (1997). *The Gift Relationship: From Human Blood to Social Policy*. New York, NY: The New Press.

Tomori, Cecilia. (2016). *Nighttime Breastfeeding: An American Cultural Dilemma*. New York, NY: Berghahn Books.

Tomori, Cecilia and Kate Boyer. (2019). "Domestic Geographies of Parental and Infant (Co-)Becomings: Home-Space, Nighttime Breastfeeding, and Parent–Infant Sleep." *Annals of the American Association of Geographers* 109(4):1172–87.

Tomori, Cecilia, Aunchalee E. L. Palmquist and Sally Dowling. (2016). "Contested Moral Landscapes: Negotiating Breastfeeding Stigma in Breastmilk Sharing, Nighttime Breastfeeding, and Long-Term Breastfeeding in the US and the UK." *Social Science & Medicine* 168:178–85.

Torres, Jennifer M. (2014). "Medicalizing to Demedicalize: Lactation Consultants and the (De)Medicalization of Breastfeeding." *Social Science & Medicine* 100:159–66.

Torres, Jennifer M. C. (2015). "Families, Markets, and Medicalization: The Role of Paid Support for Childbirth and Breastfeeding." *Qualitative Health Research* 25(7):899–911.

Totenberg, Nina. (2013). "Supreme Court OKs Discounted Resale of 'Gray Market' Goods." *All Things Considered*, NPR [Podcast]. https://www.npr.org/sections/thetwo-way/2013/03/19/174757355/supreme-court-oks-discounted-resale-of-gray-market-goods

Twine, France Winddance. (2017). "The Fertility Continuum: Racism, Bio-Capitalism and Post-Colonialism in the Transnational Surrogacy Industry." In M. Davies (ed) *Babies for Sale? Transnational Surrogacy, Human Rights and the Politics of Reproduction*. London: Zed Books, pp. 105–22.

United States Department of Labor. (2018). *Employment Characteristics of Families – 2017*. Bureau of Labor Statistics, www.bls.gov/news.release/pdf/famee.pdf

USFDA (United States Food and Drug Administration). (2010). "Use of Donor Human Milk." USFDA, www.fda.gov/ScienceResearch/SpecialTopics/PediatricTherapeuticsResearch/ucm235203.htm.

Updegrove, Kimberly. (2013). "Nonprofit Human Milk Banking in the United States." *Journal of Midwifery & Women's Health* 58(5):502–8.

Van Amsterdam, Noortje. (2015). "Othering the 'Leaky Body': An Autoethnographic Story about Expressing Breast Milk in the Workplace." *Culture and Organization* 21(3):269–87.

Van Esterik, Penny. (1989). *Beyond the Breast-Bottle Controversy*. New Brunswick, NJ: Rutgers University Press.

Van Esterik, Penny. (1996). "Expressing Ourselves: Breast Pumps." *Journal of Human Lactation* 12(4):273–74.

Van Esterik, Penny. (2002). "Contemporary Trends in Infant Feeding Research." *Annual Review of Anthropology* 31:257–278.

Waggoner, Miranda R. (2011). "Monitoring Milk and Motherhood: Lactation Consultants and the Dilemmas of Breastfeeding Advocacy." *International Journal of Sociology of the Family* (2011):153–71.

Waldby, Catherine. (2002). "Stem Cells, Tissue Cultures and the Production of Biovalue." *Health* 6(3):305–23.

Waldby, Catherine and Robert Mitchell. (2006). *Tissue Economies: Blood, Organs, and Cell Lines in Late Capitalism*. Durham, NC: Duke University Press.

Walker, Marsha and Leah S. Aldridge. (2017). "The Road to Licensure of the IBCLC." *Clinical Lactation* 8(2):53–8.

Wall, Glenda. (2001). "Moral Constructions of Motherhood in Breastfeeding Discourse." *Gender & Society* 15(4):592–610.

Wan, Elise W.-X., Kaye Davey, Madhu Page-Sharp, Peter E. Hartmann, Karen Simmer and Kenneth F. Ilett. (2008). "Dose-Effect Study of Domperidone as a Galactagogue in Preterm Mothers with Insufficient Milk Supply, and its Transfer into Milk." *British Journal of Clinical Pharmacology* 66(2):283–9.

Wasko, M. McLure and Samer Faraj. (2000). " 'It is What One Does': Why People Participate and Help Others in Electronic Communities of Practice." *The Journal of Strategic Information Systems* 9(2–3):155–73.

Wenger, Etienne. (1999). *Communities of Practice: Learning, Meaning, Identity*. Cambridge: Cambridge University Press.

Wenger. (2010). "Communities of Practice and Social Learning Systems: The Career of a Concept." In Chris Blackmore (ed) *Social Learning Systems and Communities of Practice*. London: Springer, pp. 179–98.

Wenger, Etienne C. and William M. Snyder. (2000). "Communities of Practice: The Organizational Frontier." *Harvard Business Review* 78(1):139–46.

WHO (World Health Organization). (2002). "Global Strategy on Infant and Young Child Feeding." WHO, http://apps.who.int/gb/archive/pdf_files/WHA55/ea5515.pdf?ua=1

Wilson, Kristin J. (2018). *Others' Milk: The Potential of Exceptional Breastfeeding*. New Brunswick, NJ: Rutgers University Press.

Winkelman, Warren J. and Chun Wei Choo. (2003). "Provider-Sponsored Virtual Communities for Chronic Patients: Improving Health Outcomes through Organizational Patient-Centred Knowledge Management." *Health Expectations* 6(4):352–8.

Wolf, Jacqueline. (1999). " 'Mercenary Hirelings' or 'a Great Blessing'? Doctors' and Mothers' Conflicted Perceptions of Wet Nurses and the Ramifications of Infant Feeding in Chicago, 1871–1961." *Journal of Social History* 33(1):97–120.

Wolf, Joan B. (2007). "Is Breast Really Best? Risk and Total Motherhood in the National Breastfeeding Awareness Campaign." *Journal of Health Politics, Policy and Law* 32(4):595–636.

Wolf, Joan B. (2010). *Is Breast Best?: Taking on the Breastfeeding Experts and the New High Stakes of Motherhood*. New York, NJ: New York University Press.

Wright, James D. and Amy M. Donley. (2011). *Poor and Homeless in the Sunshine State: Down and out in Theme Park Nation*. New Brunswick, NJ: Transaction Publishers.

Wuthnow, Robert. (1993). "Altruism and Sociological Theory." *Social Service Review* 67(3):344–57.

Zizzo, Gabriella. (2011). "'Donor Breast Milk is a Product from the Hospital, Not Somebody': Disassociation in Contemporary Breast Milk Banking." *Outskirts* 24.

Index

Note: Figures are indicated by italicized page references, bold indicates tables